ABIGAIL JAMES

THE
GLOW PLAN

Face massage for happy,
healthy skin in 4 weeks

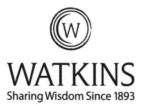

WATKINS
Sharing Wisdom Since 1893

This book is for my big brother Simon and little sister Lizzie,
you inspire me in more ways than you can ever imagine.

The Glow Plan
Abigail James

First published in the UK and USA in 2022 by
Watkins, an imprint of Watkins Media Limited
Unit 11, Shepperton House, 83–93 Shepperton Road
London N1 3DF

enquiries@watkinspublishing.com

Publisher: Fiona Robertson
Commissioning Editor: Anya Hayes
Assistant Editor: Brittany Willis
Head of Design: Karen Smith
Senior Designer: Kate Cromwell
Photographer: Katrina Lipska
Illustrations: Alice Claire Coleman and Kate Cromwell
Production: Uzma Taj

A CIP record for this book is available from the British Library

ISBN: 978-1-78678-595-4

10 9 8 7 6 5 4 3 2 1

Printed in the United Kingdom by TJ Books

www.watkinspublishing.com

CONTENTS

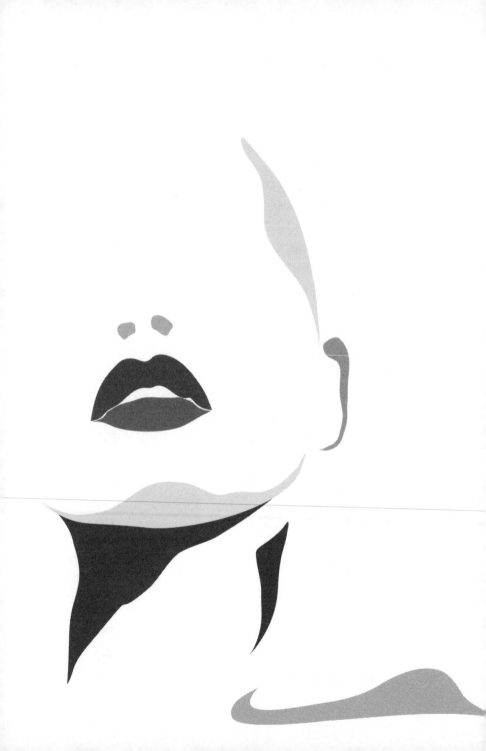

Introduction

Welcome to the Glow Plan! This book is for you if you lack energy, you never seem to have enough time for yourself, you suffer from niggling health problems – and know that all of this is affecting your skin. Perhaps your complexion has lost its glow. Maybe you've noticed a few extra lines and wrinkles. Perhaps you're tired of those dark under-eye circles. Or maybe you just want to step off the daily hamster wheel and gain the headspace you need to make better choices for yourself and your skin.

If you simply want to dial up your wellbeing and get glowing skin, you're in the right place. This plan is dedicated to addressing what your mind and body need to feel radiant, vibrant and youthful – at every age.

The focus of the Glow Plan is daily facial massage. I've been specializing in facial massage for decades – long before it became a social-media craze! Having trained professionally in a wide variety of techniques and methodologies – and performed massage on thousands of faces in my clinic – I can tell you that it's much more than just a fad. It's been an ongoing passion of mine throughout my career and I'm thrilled to have the opportunity to share my exclusive facial-massage exercises with you, so you can discover just how transformative it is too. This is your step-by-step, day-by-day plan to help you feel your most beautiful self – and really glow!

GLOW [verb] *to look attractive because you are happy and healthy*

What's Different about the Glow Plan?

There are thousands of books about skincare out there. So, what's different about this one? As an aesthetician with more than sixteen years' experience, I'm a huge believer in great skincare products and treatments. However, choosing the right products, understanding the labels and personalizing your routine is only one piece of the puzzle. To get and maintain glowing skin as we age, we need to look at the complete picture of our physical and mental wellbeing.

As a woman in my mid-forties (at the time of writing), I know this from personal experience. But this plan spans more broadly than that. During my career, I've treated everyone from teenagers to those in their seventies and beyond. This experience has given me a unique insight not simply into how our skin ages, but why. I've been able to map common causes, symptoms and ways of addressing lines, wrinkles, loss of firmness, dryness, adult acne, rosacea and generally lacklustre skin that has lost its glow.

The Glow Plan will address many facets of physical and mental wellbeing that play into the health and youthfulness of our skin. We'll explore the quality of your sleep, diet, gut health, exercise and hormones. We'll even look at how long you spend sitting at your desk, whether you live in a polluted environment, how much time you spend in nature and what supplements you may need to add into your daily routine. Naturally, we'll also address the marketing spin around skincare products, weed out anything you're using that's not working for your skin and discover how to select the right active ingredients for you.

And let's not forget your mental and emotional health, which has a symbiotic relationship with the quality of your skin. Stress and anxiety trigger our nervous system and a cascade of chemical processes that affect our skin on a cellular level, causing inflammation, collagen breakdown and accelerated ageing. Likewise, when our skin looks and feels dull, dry, saggy, sensitive and patchy, our confidence tends to drop. That inner critic shouts louder, and we enter a vicious cycle of negativity.

The Glow Plan is your opportunity to break the cycle and form new habits that benefit all aspects of your wellbeing. My wish for you is that by the end of the plan, you feel happier, have a sense of what "beautiful" means to you and know what you need to do to cultivate that inner and outer glow.

What Do I Mean by "Ageing Well"?

Ageing is part of life – and one that we should embrace. For years, women in particular have been subjected to a social narrative that tells them ageing is "bad". I believe this narrative is changing, but there's still a long way to go.

So, when I talk about ageing well, I don't mean you should conform to social pressure. This is about doing what's best for you as an individual – at a cellular, physical, emotional and intellectual level. It's about maintaining good health, finding balance and retraining our over-taxed brains to be more calm and mindful, so we can relish the joy of life and look and feel our best.

Happiness, health and how our skin looks in the mirror are all inextricably linked. Our skin is part of our identity, and as we age, we don't need to hide away or lose our sense of self. Instead, we can nurture our inner confidence, get radiant skin — and feel better than ever. Whatever your age, you can still have healthy skin that's full of life. This is what I mean by ageing well.

> **"Ageing doesn't mean giving up on style and individuality; it doesn't mean abandoning fashion and living in comfy slippers and flannel knickers"** - Twiggy

My Story

Like many women, hormonal changes have shaped my life and wellbeing. I had my first child at the age of twenty-three and suffered from the first of two episodes of postnatal depression. I've been on and off antidepressants for much of my adult life. This is not uncommon, and I have learned it's not anything to be ashamed of. If we had a physical ailment we would not question taking medication to support it! These days, I'm feeling the effects of an early menopause and the related effects on my body, skin and self-confidence.

I tell you all this because no one's life is without challenge. Yet, if there's one thing I've learnt over the decades, it's that we have a huge amount of power to change the narrative, overcome challenges and restore that inner glow. So, how did I do this?

In my twenties, I developed a passion for beauty and skincare. Juggling three small children, I trained as a beauty therapist at night school. I was hooked from the very first class. I loved learning about the intricacies of the human body; about ancient therapies and futuristic science. Since then, I've trained in many face and massage techniques, qualified as a yoga instructor and added many advanced aesthetic methods along the way. I've designed treatments for luxury global hotels and skincare brands, worked with celebrities, presented on QVC, run my own clinics and am proud to have built an online community of fellow skin and wellness enthusiasts on Instagram, YouTube and my blog and newsletter list, abigailjames.com.

It's this combination of formal training, hands-on experience and learning how to overcome obstacles within my own life that is the heart of the Glow Plan. This plan is for everyone – and it works.

What's All the Fuss about Facial Massage?

My years of training and working with clients in-clinic have given me a passion for professional treatments. From peels to LED, skin needling, radiofrequency, HIFU, light-based treatments with IPL and lasers, the technology means you really can get fantastic results.

Feeling beautiful is key. I believe that everyone can grow that inner radiance – no matter what your budget, ethnicity, age or lifestyle. The most important thing about the Glow Plan is not how much money you spend but how much energy you invest in yourself.

This book also delves into facial massage. Based on my training in Swedish and sports massage, facial reflexology, myofascial release, Thai, Ayurvedic and Indian face massage, to name just a few, we'll explore facial anatomy and the mechanics behind skin ageing.

Throughout the four-week plan in the second half of the book, I'll be giving you facial workouts with step-by-step instructions to help restore your skin's radiance and work on target areas such as your neck, jawline, cheeks, crow's feet and forehead lines, along with some lifestyle tips to help you along the way.

There is no magic bullet. Think of the four-week plan as a new way of life: you're learning new techniques and exercises which will set your skin up to look more toned, lifted and vibrant for the rest of your life. Persevere, and I promise you, you'll see results.

How to Use This Book

Any way you want! The first part of the book is about empowering yourself with the knowledge you need to look beyond the latest "miracle cream" and start truly understanding what your skin, mind and body need to thrive. You can read it chapter by chapter, or you can dip in and out of this section and get going on the four-week plan right away.

The Glow Plan is not about seeking perfection. Making a change is hard. Life is busy; maybe you have a demanding job, are juggling kids and work, are reaching or going through the menopause, or are simply overwhelmed by the constant mental overload that comes from social media and a twenty-four-hour news cycle.

Modern life tends to suck up time with things that do us no good at all. This book is here to hold your hand as you learn to break these habits and learn new, beneficial ones. The breathwork, journalling, movement practices and meditation are all there to support you along the way.

You'll also find my little black book of experts, supplement brands, skincare and make-up ranges that I rely on to keep me ageing well in the resources section at the end of the book.

Even by buying this book, you're committing to your wellbeing. You're already on the path to feeling great and getting glowing skin. I wish you good luck on your journey – remember to enjoy the ride and have fun! If it can work for me, it can definitely work for you too.

Share with me on Instagram: abigailjames1

Love, Abigail x

1

Mental Wellness

Mind, Body & Skin

Mental wellness is a subject that's close to my heart because it's been a life-long journey. I experienced my first panic attacks in my late teens and stress has always felt part of my adult life. I suffered with postnatal depression after the birth of my first child at the age of twenty-three, and again after my third at thirty.

My father taught me breathing and relaxation techniques in my teens, and arranged for me to see a hypnotherapist and acupuncturist. For someone with an old-school, religious viewpoint on life he was immensely holistic in his treatment of and attitude toward the mind. I had no idea at the time he was embedding in me a mindfulness practice which would support me throughout my life, open my eyes to many forms of therapy and enable me to support my children as well as many others.

Sometimes we need to disconnect to reconnect.

Working as a facialist and therapist for over twenty years, I have seen first-hand how powerful the mind/skin connection is. This is something I have always been very aware of. Whether it's a challenging situation that crops up out of the blue or something more long term, when our mental wellness is fragile or we are experiencing stress, we have a tendency to push through and begin to feel overwhelmed. We can find ourselves stuck in a self-perpetuating cycle of anxiety and negativity. It's often not until something gives that we finally seek help.

Someone might find me as a facialist because of a skin condition they are experiencing, and on many occasions we need to support the mind as part of the cure. Mental health can be one of the more challenging aspects of skin health to tackle; delving into emotions and finding support mechanisms is no quick fix but it is often a key part of the jigsaw.

Until recently, medical professionals have generally viewed linking mental health and the skin as a bit whimsical. We are all very familiar with complimenting a friend on their "holiday glow" when they seem particularly happy and relaxed, or commenting that someone has gone "grey overnight" after experiencing a sudden tragedy – but this is anecdotal, not scientific.

There is, however, a growing body of scientific research that connects our mental wellbeing with how our skin functions and looks. This understanding is timely, given that mental health challenges are becoming more and more prevalent. It doesn't have to be the all-encompassing mental breakdown – it can be the daily challenges, including work and family stress, career issues, financial worries, illness, relationship concerns and all sorts of decision-making challenges. Not to mention the fast pace and "always on" culture of our lives, a never-ending (and often depressing) news cycle and the expectations and huge pressures social media brings to all of us to look or be a certain way. We feel like we need to fit a specific ideal and have it all sorted. For most of us, that's far from the case; we are winging it and stumbling through the journey of life!

Social media can have such positive influence on life, giving voices to those with something good to share. But it is also a breeding ground for insecurities, fuelling imposter syndrome and feeling like you're failing in life.

In this chapter, I want to explore the link between mental wellness and skin and why it's a key factor to ageing well. Then we'll work through some simple daily practices to help combat stress, feel happier and healthier, recover our glow and, of course, age better.

Stress and Ageing – What's Happening Beneath the Surface?

When we talk about "worry lines" or "going as white as a sheet", it's clear that our emotions really do show up on our skin. Yet, as with most things, this reality is more complex than something that's just skin deep.

When we're stressed, blood flow is directed internally to our essential organs and in particular to our muscles so that we can run or fight off the immediate danger – the fight-or-flight response. As a result, there's less blood travelling to our skin (which is why colour literally drains from someone's face when they're in shock). The supply of nutrients the blood delivers to our skin decreases, cell turnover is compromised and healing slows. When we put that into the context of our constant state of modern-day stress, that's a regular impact on how our body is naturally supporting the skin.

Stress can also alter the production of collagen and directly impact the elasticity and radiance of our skin. The more stressed you are, the older you're likely to look. It might not be showing on the skin just yet, but it can catch up with you over the years. The good news is that with more knowledge, we can begin to rebalance the ageing process – and take a more positive approach to ageing.

Stress and DNA

Stress affects our telomeres. These are small elements that sit at the ends of DNA strands to stop them fraying, rather like the ends of shoelaces. These DNA "tips" protect our chromosomes, but stress can cause them to "unravel" or "fray". Over time, these telomeres get shorter and shorter, which accelerates the ageing process. So, stress isn't just an emotional issue. Just like genetics, diet and our external environment, the impact of stress on our health and mortality are now the subject of serious scientific enquiry.

A few years ago, a study revealed that among a group of fifty-eight perimenopausal women, the cellular age of those who were highly stressed was ten years older than their actual age.[1] Imagine this effect compounding over a lifetime, and we can begin to see just how much stress directs whether we age well.

Stress and the skin barrier

"Skin barrier function" has become a bit of a buzz-phrase in the skincare industry since brands began formulating products specifically designed to repair and strengthen it. If the barrier function is happy then everything else under the surface can skip along more happily too.

The skin barrier acts as a vital line of defence against external factors such as chemicals, pollution and UV radiation (I will cover these in more detail in Chapter 4). As well as keeping harmful elements out, it also helps retain your skin's natural oils and moisture, maintaining a balance known as homeostasis. When the skin barrier is functioning well, your skin looks healthy, hydrated, firm and glowing. When it's unable to behave as it should, your skin can become dry, dull and dehydrated and develop breakouts, and over time result in irritation, redness and sensitivity. All things we don't want for the skin and issues that can accelerate the visible appearance of the ageing process.

Research tells us that stress hormones compromise our skin barrier function by decreasing the skin's natural lipids (fats) and structural proteins that keep it healthy and resilient. Stress can also reduce hydration levels and increase trans-epidermal water loss.[2] Our skin literally has stress written all over it.

Stress and the skin microbiome

The link between gut health, overall wellbeing and mental wellness has attracted an increasing amount of scientific discovery recently. I will cover gut health – and how to optimize it – in Chapter 5. What's interesting to note here is that the skin – like the gut – has its own microbiome: an eco-system of living organisms that's unique to every one of us. Stress – along with our internal and external lifestyle and environmental factors – can upset the delicate balance of these organisms, compromising the skin's ability to renew, repair and remain resilient and youthful. Reducing stress levels and using the right type of skincare can help rebalance the skin microbiome and recover our natural glow.

Stress and eczema, psoriasis and dermatitis

If you developed one of these conditions during adulthood, you're not alone. Around 1.9 billion people worldwide suffer from these types of inflammatory skin conditions – and like acne, they're on the rise.[3] Again, stress comes into play. Too much of the stress hormone cortisol can suppress our immune system and trigger an inflammatory response, to which people with eczema and dry skin conditions are already particularly susceptible.

Stress and acne

Spots and acne have long been associated with the disrupted hormones of teenagers. During my career I have seen an epidemic of adult acne among people of all ages. The *Journal of the American Academy of Dermatology* suggests that as many as 53 per cent of women aged twenty-five and above now have some facial acne!

Of all the many causes of acne, studies demonstrate a strong correlation between severe stress and adult acne and I can vouch for this from the clients I see in clinic. It's often those with the highest stress lives that have the most challenging skin.

Stress triggers the release of adrenal hormones and substances that may enlarge sebaceous (oil) glands, increase the number of these glands and stimulate oil production. All of which are primary causes of acne. As stress can limit our body's ability to repair itself, it can also lead to more severe and prolonged acne scarring.

The impact skin issues can have on your mental wellbeing is huge. Acne and eczema might not be life-threatening conditions within themselves, however, bearing the physical marks of inflammation and breakouts has been shown to dramatically impact people's self-esteem, leading to low moods, depression, social anxiety, days off work and even self-imposed isolation. The more our mental health suffers, the greater the impact on our skin's health and the worse we feel about ourselves.

A NOTE ON
SKIN-FLAMMAGEING

There's another type of inflammation that's worth considering when thinking about how we can age better. This type of inflammation is known as "inflammageing", or (in direct relation to the skin) "skin-flammageing". It refers to inflammation that takes place at a cellular level.

Acute inflammation, which could manifest as redness, swelling and a rash, is usually triggered by a physiological assault on the skin – like burning or cutting yourself. In contrast, inflammageing refers to chronic and low-grade inflammation that remains undetected for many years. It increases as we age, and in turn, accelerates the ageing process. It's generally caused by free radicals, from things like smoking, an imbalanced diet, sun exposure, pollution and (of course) STRESS. This type of inflammation sets off a domino effect of negative responses inside our body.

The 'inflammatory cascade', as the chain reaction of responses is known, can cause the body to produce more of the enzyme hyaluronidase. This enzyme breaks down naturally occurring hyaluronic acid, something that helps our skin retain its youthful vibrancy, plumpness and dewiness.

Inflammation also affects fibroblasts. Located within the skin's connective tissue, they're responsible for producing collagen and helping to maintain the skin's structure. When their function is impaired, collagen begins to break down. Over time, this low-level, chronic inflammation can cause the skin to become dry, dull and uneven in tone. Its texture becomes less smooth, we notice our skin is less firm, and lines and wrinkles begin to appear and set in.

Psychodermatology – Treating the Mind to Save the Skin

In 1857, English dermatologist and surgeon William James Erasmus Wilson wrote the book *On Diseases of the Skin,* in which he described a phenomenon he called "skin neurosis".[4]

As we've seen throughout this chapter, our mind, skin and the rate at which we age are intricately linked. William James Erasmus Wilson was ahead of his time because the modern-day field of psychodermatology is still a relatively new one. As you can probably guess, it merges the two medical specialties of psychiatry and dermatology to both prevent and treat a whole host of skin issues.

Psychodermatology involves looking at the complex interplay between the neurological, immunological, cutaneous (relating to skin sensitivity and our ability to detect changes in pressure, temperature, vibrations and pain) and endocrine (hormone) systems. It addresses the mind/skin connection in three main ways: by looking at skin problems that are affected by our emotional state, by understanding how psychological skin disorders negatively impact our mental health and by analyzing psychiatric disorders that manifest themselves via the skin.

What's perhaps most interesting is that techniques such as hypnosis, guided meditation, cognitive behavioural therapy and other forms of psychotherapy can not only help alleviate the mental angst associated with skin conditions but can also increase the efficacy of topical treatments! In one study, people who listened to a mindfulness meditation programme while undergoing phototherapy treatment for rosacea needed 40 per cent less exposure to ultraviolet light than others.[5]

Experts are working on a variety of ways to improve our emotional response to skin issues such as acne, eczema and – of course – ageing. It's easy to fall into the comparison game; scrolling through Instagram is enough to make even the most self-confident woman feel like she has too many wrinkles or her face is sagging before her time and doesn't match some impossible standard of (usually heavily filtered) perfection.

All of this is counterintuitive, because as we've seen, the more stress we experience, the greater the impact on our ageing process. While I'm a huge believer in skincare products that are formulated with good-quality ingredients, there is no one magic potion. By relying on topical products to treat our skin, boost our glow and help us remain youthful for longer, we're treating the symptom – not the cause. So, let's change some habits and start ageing better – this is where my skin glow plan comes into play.

The relationship we have with ourselves is the most important relationship of our lives

Mindset Tools for Mental Wellness

Shifting the narrative

In the next section, I'll share tools and techniques I try to use in my life to change my mindset, feel happier and reduce stress. There are no hard and fast rules here, but consistency is key. Creating and sticking to a routine of healthy habits has been proven to lessen stress and anxiety, improve quality of sleep, help us feel more in control and enable us to make better choices for our overall health and wellbeing.[6] Try and build these habits into your life by making a plan to do them at roughly the same time each day.

Affirmations

An affirmation is a sentence or statement that can help you overcome a negative belief.

They might conjure up images of looking in the mirror and telling yourself how great you are – over and over again. Affirmations in this form might feel awkward, to say the least. Yet, science might persuade you otherwise.

MRI evidence suggests that when people practise self-affirmation, certain neural pathways increase. This means that positive self-affirmations can help shape (or shift) our view of ourselves. Most of us walk around telling ourselves we're not good enough, not doing enough or don't look the right way. Far from being helpful, this can become a self-perpetuating cycle in which our self-esteem gets progressively lower. Affirmations can help us feel more capable and resilient in the face of challenge, help boost our self-esteem, lower stress levels, reduce anxiety to promote better sleep and give us a more positive outlook on life.

We speak to ourselves more than we do anyone else, and often we are the most critical voices we will ever hear. We should speak to ourselves with the kindness and love we show to our best friend.

Positive affirmations help us change our internal conversation. So rather than getting caught up in negative self-talk, we replace these thought patterns with something more useful. Changing our mental narrative in this way has been shown to bring a long list of benefits, one of which is that we begin to think of our identity more flexibly – we're not "just" an employee, a mother or a good friend; we play many valuable roles in life. We are independent, kind and have so much to offer to this life.

Affirmations aren't magic, but they are effective – and do require consistency. Ideally, you should choose between one and five positive affirmations that challenge self-critical thoughts. Try and repeat them – aloud or in your head – at least once a day, if not more often. Like laughter, affirmations have been shown to release endorphins, helping us "rewire" our brain mapping and change our mindset.[7]

I have included lots of lovely affirmations throughout the plan to guide you to a more confident, positive you.

Journalling

Journalling is an old-school practice which went out of vogue with the onset of all of us being attached to a screen. However the benefits can be profound.

I started journalling when I first suffered from postnatal depression. I found myself waking in the middle of the night, head racing with a million thoughts and worries. I began writing these thoughts down in a journal I kept beside my bed to give myself the headspace I needed to sleep. I didn't make a conscious decision to "start journalling", it just felt good to do. Often the words would be frantic, not make much sense to others but that wasn't the point – simply getting your thoughts out of your head onto paper is so powerful.

People have been recording their thoughts and emotions in diaries and letters for centuries. Modern-day science tells us that the benefits of journalling stem from its ability to help us access the left side of our brain,[8] which is responsible for analytical or rational thinking (as opposed to the right side, which is involved in intuition and creativity).

Unlocking this left-brain thinking helps us gain perspective and clarity about our thoughts and emotions, rather than suppressing or allowing them to control us. Studies have shown that regular journalling can help to reduce stress and anxiety, boost our mood, improve our ability to problem-solve, meet goals – and resolve conflict. It also enables us to look back and track patterns that might have had a negative impact on our lives – or helped us through a time we found particularly challenging. If all that isn't convincing enough, some experts believe that journalling can strengthen immune cells called T-lymphocytes, reduce blood pressure and even help relieve asthma.[9]

My tips for journalling:

- Journal daily. Preferably at the same time each day, so it becomes a habit – like cleaning your teeth. Aim for somewhere between five to twenty minutes – there is no steadfast rule; this isn't intended to be a chore.

- Write freely. This is not about creating perfect prose, so write in whatever structure that works best for you without getting hung up on spelling or grammar. Whether you write about what happened in your day or something that's challenging you, try and let it flow like a stream of consciousness.

- Create a theme. This can be a helpful way of focusing your attention on a single topic each week or month. It could be happiness, anger, self-criticism – anything that feels relevant to you.

- Keep it private. This is your time to explore things that you might not otherwise feel comfortable sharing with someone else.

- Reflect without judgement. At the end of each session, give yourself a few minutes to think about any key takeaways that might be useful in your day. Don't fall into the trap of judging yourself – this is an open space to gain clarity, not an opportunity to beat yourself up.

- Journal through the good times as well as the bad. It's good to be able to go back to your journal and see how things were during the good times as well as the challenges, learn from them and appreciate them.

Gratitude

It's easy to get caught in a "woe is me" pattern of thinking. We are now led to believe we *can* have it all, and we *should* have it all. This is all very well but it doesn't leave much space for gratitude.

We live at a time when the world is at our fingertips yet it's become commonplace to want more. Setting challenges for yourself is natural and healthy. Living in a perpetual state of feeling that who you are or what you have is never enough can only breed unhappiness, resentment and a feeling that you're destined to remain unfulfilled.

We often rush through life without taking the time to notice the little things around us and there are so many ways we can shift our focus and change our outlook.

Practising gratitude is not about mindlessly reeling off a list of good things in your life. It's about feeling it, connecting emotionally with the people and things that add value, including the small, simple aspects of life – and picturing what your life would be like without them. It's easy to imagine that other people's lives are perfect or worry-free (believe me, they are not!). It's worth remembering that for every one of the things you take for granted, there is most definitely someone else who would love what you have.

A study by the University of California showed that after ten weeks of practising gratitude, participants' outlook on life was noticeably more optimistic.[10] It helps shift our mindset from being disappointed, down and defeatist, to actively seeking the small things that spark in our life. The more we notice the things we're thankful for, the happier we become. We create a kind of positive feedback loop for our brain that progressively enhances our mental wellbeing over time.

There are many different ways of building gratitude into your life – we will be working on this through the weekly plan. Here are some techniques that have helped me:

- Pick a regular time each day to actively think about what makes you feel thankful. This might mean writing things down in a journal first thing in the morning, or three minutes in the bathroom instead of scrolling Instagram while on the loo. For me, it's my shower time; I crave that time to myself and do a lot of my reflection and thinking in the shower.

- Think small. It doesn't matter if it's simply a sunny day, the wifi worked well today, clean bed sheets, your new facial cleanser. Practising gratitude is about finding as many moments in the day to experience it as you can – not waiting for weeks or months for the "one big thing" that makes everything seem better.

- Feel it – don't just think it. It's almost impossible to conjure an extremely positive and very negative emotion at the same time. When you practise gratitude, really allow yourself the time to explore how a moment, thing or person made you feel.

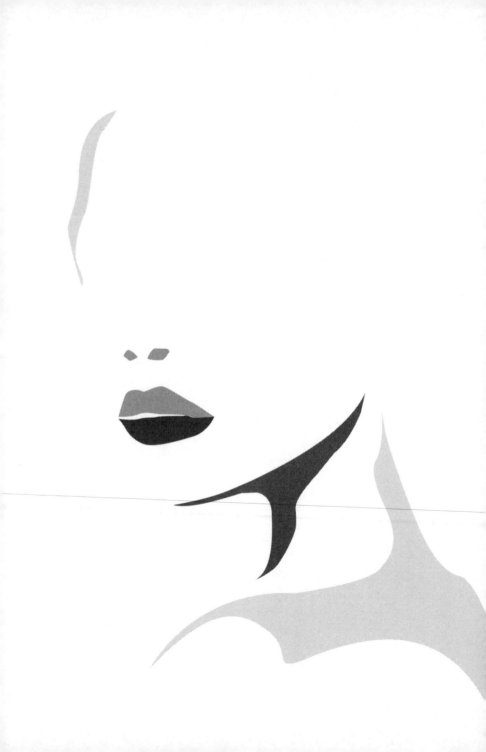

2

Sleep Wellness

Ageing Around the Clock

I am a seasoned insomniac. So much so that I feel like it's part of my DNA. Even as a child, I remember sliding into my mum's side of the bed in the early hours of the morning when I couldn't sleep. Perhaps it's why I'm fascinated by sleep. I've spent years educating myself on how we can try to optimize our sleep – and what to do when our body's screaming out for it.

We all know how difficult it is to function – mentally and physically – after a poor night's sleep. We're sluggish; we have trouble concentrating; we're grouchy and more susceptible to stress. That's before we mention the effect on our skin: puffy eyes, dark circles and a dull, lifeless complexion are all the hallmarks of a night spent tossing and turning. We may be able to get away with it when we're younger, but for most of us, this is no longer the case as we age.

The occasional bad night's sleep is one thing. Most of us tend to bounce back after some decent rest. However, sleep deprivation over a long period of time has a cumulative effect that scientists have linked to a number of physical and mental issues. So, when it comes to ageing well, understanding sleep science is an essential piece of the puzzle.

Achieving eight hours of sleep every night is easier said than done! I have spent many a night getting increasingly emotional for not being able to do something as simple as getting to sleep or staying asleep.

In modern society, sleep seems to be in crisis. Not only are sleep disorders on the rise, but it's become a kind of badge of honour to boast about how little sleep we can "get away with". We spend so much time looking at screens, and less of our day outside in natural light. We put working, train schedules and our social lives first. For many people, sleep sits at the bottom of their priority list. I would argue that this is about to change as our understanding of sleep and how it can empower us deepens.

Throughout this chapter, we'll look at how sleep can unlock mental and physical wellness. Then we'll work through some daily habits that can help improve the quality of sleep – and, of course, help you stay youthful for longer.

Why is Circadian Science so Important?

Most of us have been told to aim for around eight hours of sleep per night. Yet, circadian science – a fast-developing field of research – tells us that sleep is more complicated and individual than that. Ageing well is not just about how *much* you sleep, but *when* you sleep.

Circadian processes were mentioned in Chinese medical texts as early as the 13th century. In 2017, the Nobel Prize in Physiology or Medicine had been awarded for research into circadian genes that control our daily rhythms. Today, it's thought that there are many as 351 genes that influence our individual "chronotype".[11]

Our chronotype is a genetically determined internal clock that governs our sleep and activity patterns across twenty-four hours. This clock is the reason we hear about larks and owls. If you're a lark, you're likely to rise early, be most productive before noon and sleep earlier – but not without suffering a mid-afternoon slump in alertness and productivity. Owls wake late, sleep late – and might not even get going until around 4pm. Chronobiologists (scientists who study sleep patterns) estimate that around 80 per cent of us actually sit somewhere between these two extremes, rising and sleeping at more moderate times.[12] I used to be an owl; however, over the years I've changed into more of a lark.

So, why is our circadian rhythm so important? Our circadian clock controls the timings of every organ system and bodily process. When it suffers long-term disruption – by work schedules, our diet or watching box sets late into the night – we increase our risk of allergies, cardiovascular disease, gut disorders, obesity, premature ageing and so much more.[13] The activity of the circadian system is the reason why you're more likely to suffer a heart attack at 6.30am than any other time of day or night![14]

I know many people including myself find they wake up at the same time every morning – this can all be connected to our natural circadian processes. Find your body's natural sleep/wake cycle, then try to stick to it. Consistency – not simply quantity – is vital when it comes to optimizing our sleep.

Sleep, Happiness and Success

Sleep has the power to limit, or unlock, enhanced brain function and mental wellbeing. In Chapter 1, we looked at how stress can affect how well we age. People who sleep less than eight hours a night report higher levels of stress.[15] There's also a strong correlation between insomnia, anxiety and stress.[16]

On the flip side, tuning into your body's circadian rhythm and getting good-quality sleep can have a hugely uplifting impact on your mood. After just a single good night's sleep, you can feel the difference: you're more refreshed, the brain switches back on and you generally feel calmer. The cumulative benefits of good sleep, night after night, are even more compelling. Research shows that good sleepers are more likely to be optimistic, motivated and perform better in their careers – so much for politicians and FTSE100 leaders surviving on four hours a night.[17] And for my many years juggling a career and being a single parent of three!

If you're already a good sleeper, this may all come as music to your ears. If, like me, you've spent hours wondering whether it's better to count sheep, clean the house or give up on sleep entirely, there is good news. By better understanding sleep, we can learn to reset our internal clock and, ultimately, age better.

Sleep and Ageing – Your Skin Has a Circadian Rhythm Too

Most of us recognize that there's a link between the quality of our sleep and the appearance of our skin, because we see it with our own eyes. Look in the mirror after a sleepless night and you're likely to see eye bags, dark circles, fine lines more pronounced, red patches and a generally lifeless face looking back at you. Anyone who suffers from conditions like eczema and acne will know how much worse they can be after a night of sleep disruption.

Yet, as well as the day-to-day effect sleeplessness has on our skin, it also directly impacts how fast and well we age over time. Research shows that just one bad night's sleep can make our cells age faster.[18] Just imagine what many months, years or even a lifetime of poor sleep can do! If we want to age well, we've got to sleep well.

Sleep and repair

Our skin cells have their own clocks, and keep their own time.[19] During the day, our skin is in defence mode as it works to protect us from external aggressors like UV light and pollution (I will cover this in Chapter 4). At night, our skin enters recovery mode as it repairs the damage from the day. Between the hours of 11pm and 4am, cell production can double as human growth hormones are secreted to encourage regeneration and repair.[20] The antioxidant and anti-inflammatory sleep hormone melatonin, which peaks at around 2am, also protects our skin from free-radical damage. When our sleep/wake cycle is imbalanced and these processes are impaired, tissue repair is compromised and our skin becomes more sensitive and susceptible to ageing.

One study found that late-night eating could put our skin at greater risk of sun damage during the day. The reason being that midnight snacking brings the circadian clock backward (to a regular evening dinner time), thereby delaying the activation of an enzyme involved in UV protection come morning.[21]

Sleep and cortisol

We know that when we sleep, we perspire, which accelerates the body's natural detoxification process. When this process stalls, the skin quickly becomes clogged, dull and prone to breakouts. A lack of sleep causes the stress hormone cortisol to be released. As mentioned in Chapter 1, cortisol triggers an inflammatory response within the skin that can cause sensitivity, flare-ups of skin conditions such as acne and trigger the breakdown of collagen.

Sleep and collagen

We know that collagen helps to support the skin's structure. Poor -quality sleep can impact how effectively it's produced, both by limiting the production of human growth hormone (which stimulates cell production) and by changing our body's natural immune response.[22] Over time, our skin loses its youthful elasticity and begins to sag or develop fine lines and wrinkles.

Sleep and the skin barrier

Research shows that in weakening the skin barrier function, a lack of sleep can make us more vulnerable to conditions like eczema, rosacea and psoriasis.[23] A weak skin barrier can also result in increased trans-epidermal water loss (when moisture evaporates from the skin's surface). As a result, our skin can become dry, irritated and fine lines and wrinkles may become more prominent.

Sleep and blood vessels

Of all the skin issues that bother people, dark circles are usually near the top of the list. Although caused by myriad factors, sleep quality is not only an important one but unlike genetics, hormones and our external environment, it's one that we're able to influence. When we don't sleep well, the blood vessels beneath the thin skin around the eyes can dilate. The more blood flows through these vessels, the more visible it becomes. This is what causes those purple shadows in the hollow of our lower-eye contour. Fluid can also accumulate and leak out into the skin tissues, which is why we often look puffy and swollen after a particularly bad night's sleep.

A NOTE ON
SLEEP & GUT HEALTH

Until recently, a connection between our gut and sleep quality might have felt tenuous. Yet, the field of microbiome science has advanced rapidly, and good gut health is now thought to play a vital role in our overall health, skin and in the quality of our sleep.

Research by the University of Tsukuba in Japan found that a healthy gut microbiome (the community of bacteria and fungi living within the gut) may help stabilize our sleep/wake cycle. It does this by helping to create important chemical brain messengers like serotonin (the chemical precursor to melatonin) and dopamine, the hormone that helps us feel more alert.[24]

We know that what we eat can influence the eco-system of micro-organisms within our gut.[25] So, to sleep well and age better, we need to eat smart. We'll cover what to eat – and when – to optimize gut health at the end of this chapter.

I know that when my diet is healthier – lots of veg and lean meat, cutting out biscuits and coffee, etc. – my overall energy levels are so much better, and adding in a daily probiotic has been a game changer.

Setting Yourself Up for a Good Sleep

The term "sleep hygiene" often crops up on social media. It's basically a posh phrase for a good bedtime routine by reducing things that might keep you awake and getting into better habits that support sleep.

When we're children (or when we *have* children), we tend to live by an almost unshakeable bedtime routine. When my kids were younger it was essential, not just for them but for me as well. In the evening we'd eat, have a bath, relax with a book or bedtime story, lights off by a certain time and done. As adults, this routine gets out of whack, or even thrown out of the window completely, for any number of things: increased time on mobiles and screens, late working hours and night shifts, partying, early morning meetings and long commutes. It's easy to fall into the mindset that we don't have time to sleep, which is just crazy! The less we sleep, the less we *can* sleep. So, sleeplessness becomes a self-perpetuating cycle.

I know as a hedonistic teenager on a night out I had to be the last man standing, often not going to sleep at all – I had no idea I was setting myself up for a lifetime of more sleep issues. Now a good night for me is in bed by 9pm.

The most important thing is that if you feel tired at 9pm, go with it. There's no rule about having to stay up until 11pm – so don't ignore what your body clock is trying to tell you. Try and sleep at the same time every night and wake at the same time each morning. Ideally we would resist the weekend lie-in because even a one-hour difference can throw your circadian clock out of whack. I often wake at the same time on the weekend but enjoy lying in bed for longer, reading the papers with hot tea, so I am physically awake but also still enjoying the time to relax.

Your Better Sleep Toolkit

In this section, I'll share some of the sleep tips and techniques that have worked for me. As with everything, repetition and routine are key for success.

Light and sleep

While our circadian rhythm is governed by our brains, it's also affected by cues from our external environment. Light is one such cue. Typically, exposure to natural daylight helps us sleep earlier and get a better night's rest. Researchers have found that light wavelengths at sunrise and sunset have the greatest impact on the brain centres that regulate our circadian clock, mood and alertness.[26]

One reason why many of us have trouble sleeping is that we spend our day working inside, so have limited exposure to natural light. At night time, we're bombarded by artificial light – from light bulbs, smartphones and televisions. Blue light from LED screens tricks our brain into thinking it doesn't need to release melatonin and pushes our sleep/wake cycle back.[27]

It's easier said than done. I have had many days when I'm in clinic, arriving early in the morning, fresh off the Tube, and not leaving before 8pm when it's dark outside. I *know* this is not good for my health. So I try and get outside for at least twenty to thirty minutes every day – as soon after waking as possible. Ideally, you'd also dim your lights and avoid screens for at least three hours before you want to go to sleep. If that feels like an impossible task, lights that harness the latest findings in circadian science are now available to help us reset our rhythm and sleep better. Or you can wear light-protecting glasses.

Eating for sleep

Almost every cell in our body runs by a clock. Our digestive system is no different. According to chrononutrition (a way of eating in accordance with your circadian rhythm), we're primed to eat earlier in the day, when the sun is shining, and fast when it gets dark, which is almost the total opposite of what we generally do. Once melatonin production has begun, the body can struggle to produce enough insulin to digest a heavy meal. So, it's better to eat earlier (at least two hours before bedtime) and lighter in the evening, which isn't half as sociable as we might like. Try to finish eating by 9pm at the very latest. I am still a fan of eating around 6–6.30pm as I always used to with the children when they were young.

Nutrients to include in your evening meal

- **Vitamin B6:** this vital nutrient supports the body's melatonin production. Tuna, wild salmon, chicken, potatoes, whole grains, bananas, prunes, cooked spinach and sunflower seeds are all rich sources.

- **Magnesium:** many women in particular are deficient in this sleep-aiding mineral. Find it in fish, almonds, leafy greens and bananas.

- **Vitamin E:** appears to help protect the brain from memory loss associated with sleep deprivation. Try upping your intake of sunflower oil, rainbow trout, almonds, Brazil nuts, pumpkin, red pepper, asparagus and avocado.

- **Tryptophan:** this nutrient helps support melatonin and serotonin production to stabilize our sleep/wake cycle. You'll find it in turkey, chicken, whole milk, eggs, tofu and oatmeal.

Good gut foods

Certain foods can influence the diversity of beneficial bacteria within our gut microbiome, which, as we've seen, could help regulate your sleep/wake cycle. These fermented and prebiotic-rich foods should be eaten during the day, rather than at night: live yoghurt, kefir, miso, kimchi, sauerkraut, tempeh, Jerusalem artichokes, leeks and onions.

Foods to avoid

Certain foods contain tyramine, an amino acid that can act as a brain stimulant. These include: aubergine, pineapple, tomato, aged cheese, cured and processed meat and citrus fruits. The cheese board at the end of a meal really is a bad idea!

For a good night's sleep, it's best to limit your intake of sugar, artificial sweeteners, caffeine, alcohol and refined carbohydrates. I've lost count of the number of nights I've lain awake and realized that I ate dark chocolate after dinner, so I tend to avoid it after 2pm.

My favourite supplements for sleep

- **Ashwagandha:** an evergreen shrub that's also known as Indian ginseng, proven to both improve sleep quality and help tackle insomnia.[28]

- **Magnesium glycinate:** often used to calm, lessen anxiety, relieve muscle tension and promote better sleep.

- **Magnolia bark:** assists with stress, anxiety and depression; the polyphenols have been found to support sleep with a sedative effect.

- **Valerian:** often referred to as "nature's Valium", this tall flowering grassland plant may improve your stress response and help you fall asleep quicker.

- **5-HTP (5-Hydroxytryptophan):** used to produce serotonin, which is converted to melatonin, to help regulate your sleep/wake cycle. It also has other mood-boosting benefits.

- **GABA (Gamma-aminobutyric acid):** an amino acid that works as a neurotransmitter within the brain. It's been shown to help you fall asleep faster, as well as improve symptoms associated with stress and fatigue.[29]

When to exercise

Exercise plays an essential role in our overall wellbeing – and affects our sleep quality. I often find when I have a sedentary day, I don't sleep so well. So, I try and incorporate some kind of movement – even if it's just a walk – into my daily routine; even better if I have broken into a sweat.

The scientific jury is still out as to whether it's better to exercise in the morning or evening. Some circadian science suggests that we should exercise around four hours after waking (as opposed to first thing in the morning when you're sleepy and your performance might be compromised) and four hours before sleeping (so as not to overstimulate your body before bedtime). That means that for most of us, lunchtime is the ideal time to work out. If you can get outside into natural daylight, that's even better. The most important thing is to find a time that you can stick to.

Meditation

Meditation is not just about sitting cross-legged and emptying your mind. It's actually the opposite; it's about focusing the mind on something quite specific, other than what's going on in your head. It would be impossible to totally empty your thoughts! Our minds are generally working overtime with to-do lists and the constant ticker tape of information. Meditation helps you to shift out of autopilot and calm the mind.

My father first taught me a form of meditation in my late teens when I was suffering from anxiety and panic attacks. I recall him getting me to lie on the sofa and focus on individual parts of my body while breathing slower. Over a decade later when I first started going to yoga classes in London, I realized it was a form of yoga nidra he was teaching me.

Meditation is a mind/body practice that has existed for millennia. There are many different types, but some things they have in common are: finding a quiet place where you won't be disturbed; focusing your attention on a word, body part, external thing like a flame, or a mantra; conscious breathwork and maintaining an open attitude to changing the state of both your mind and body.

Most people tend to turn to meditation as a means of relieving stress or anxiety. Yet, the benefits of mindfulness meditation (a practice that focuses on remaining in the present moment and releasing negative thoughts) go far beyond that. A team of Harvard scientists found that just eight weeks of mindfulness meditation increased cortical thickness in the brain's hippocampus, which governs learning and memory.[30] Another study found that practising for just four days helped reduce levels of the stress hormone cortisol, and made people feel happier.[31]

A growing body of research suggests that meditation can help manage symptoms associated with everything from asthma and depression to chronic pain, tension headaches, high blood pressure, heart disease, irritable bowel syndrome and even cancer.[32] It won't surprise you to discover that it has also been found to help improve sleep. It does so by evoking our "relaxation response" – a term coined in the 1970s to signify a deep psychological shift that's the opposite of our body's reaction to stress.[33]

A sleep meditation practice

After many sleepless nights, I began to look for a meditation technique that helps promote better sleep. I follow this thirty-minute mindfulness meditation practice, particularly if I've had a hard day or am going through a super stressful period.[34]

1. Find a comfortable position, somewhere nice and warm, either seated on a chair or lying down.

2. Close your eyes, and take a few deep breaths. Take a moment to tune into the natural rhythm of your breath. Begin to focus on the sensations of your breathing.

3. Notice where you feel your breath most distinctly. It could be on the tip of your nose, or the rise and fall of your abdomen. Wherever it is that you feel the breath, focus on the raw sensations that accompany inhaling and exhaling without trying to control it.

4. As you focus on your breath, you'll begin to notice other sensations around the body, as well as thoughts and sounds. Observe them, then come back to the breath.

5. The moment you become aware that you're thinking, either in images or words, just notice the thought. Then return to the physical sensations of breathing.

6. Now, gently shift your attention to your physical body, and let yourself ground into the surface beneath you. Notice which parts of your body feel most connected to the surface you're on. Some body parts might be easier to feel than others – so just notice this.

7. As you centre your awareness on your body, you might start to notice physical sensations. Perhaps a tingling in your palms or feet, or a sense of energy flowing through your body.

8. Notice how quickly these physical sensations come and go and the intensity with which they arise.

9. Start to consciously relax your entire body, all the way from your toes up to your head and along your arms to your fingertips. Notice any tension you're holding on to, whether it's in your neck, your jaw, your face or anywhere else.

10. What does the tension feel like? Maybe it's a heaviness, like a weight. Or maybe it's a tightness. Whatever you feel, just become aware of the physical sensation of tension in the body.

11. Now, begin to let go of that tension. Imagine taking off a heavy rucksack after a long day. Focus on shedding the heavy layers and allow your body to experience a feeling of weightlessness as you drift off to sleep.

Breathwork for better sleep

Breathing techniques have, of course, been around for centuries. Yet it's only recently that breathwork has come into its own, as several experts and studios began to offer a variety of different modalities. Each of these techniques involves consciously altering your breathing pattern to achieve a certain outcome. I came across this within my yoga teacher training.

The clue is in the "work": this is not just about involuntarily inhaling and exhaling. It's about consistently working to strengthen your diaphragm and improve your breathing patterns day after day – like a fitness routine. Not for nothing are the Navy Seals trained in breathwork to help them deal with high-pressure situations.

A regular breathwork practice can bring a whole host of physical and mental benefits – from lowering our blood pressure and increasing infection-fighting white blood cells to oxygenating our muscles and relieving tension. As 70 per cent of toxins leave the body via the lungs, it's also a vital means of detoxification. Full, diaphragmatic breathing can even help massage the intestines, helping to relieve symptoms of IBS and improve nutrient absorption.

By controlling glucose levels which impact cell ageing, breathwork can help get your skin glowing – and is even said to release a substance called "vagusstoff", which acts like a natural tranquillizer. Naturally, this makes it the perfect thing to practise before bed.

My tips for breathing well:

- Inhale through the nose silently, feeling your diaphragm and back expand softly and fully without forcing it. Inhale right to the top.

- Notice as your ribs fill with air and your lower belly expands outward.

- Your chest and upper back may rise at the peak of the inhalation.

- Exhale through your nose. Feel your belly slowly empty, your ribs deflate and your chest return to its resting position.

- Try to smooth out each round of inhalation and exhalation, so it becomes rhythmic and continually flowing with no gaps.

- Inhale for the count of five, exhale for the count of eight.

A bedtime breathwork practice

1. Lie on your stomach or on your side, whichever feels most comfortable (I like putting a pillow between my knees if I'm on my side).

2. Imagine yourself sinking into the mattress as you let all tension go.

3. If you're lying on your side, put your hand under your pillow in line with your ear. This will apply a little pressure between your ear and your pillow.

4. Bring your awareness to the space between the pillow and your hand. You should be able to hear your heartbeat.

5. Use this beat as a guide for your breathing. Breathe in through your nose for six beats, hold for two and exhale for eight.

6. Continue for as many rounds as you need. You may notice your heartbeat slows down after a while and you may even drift off mid-count.

Yoga nidra

Yoga nidra is another form of meditative practice that works by softening the body to help induce deep relaxation and put you in a sleep-like state. It hails from ancient India but has even been used by the American Army to help soldiers recover from post-traumatic stress disorder.[35] Research shows that it's a highly effective way of reducing stress and anxiety levels.[36] When performed just before bedtime, I find it helps calm my racing mind and relax any muscle tension left over from the day.

This is a method I use a lot, especially those nights I can't switch my brain off; it's a really simple one to follow on your own once you know the process.

1. Bring your awareness to your right foot. Then focus on your fifth toe, fourth toe, third toe, second toe and big toe. Notice the sensations around your toes.

2. Bring your awareness to the sole of your foot, heel, inner ankle and outer ankle. Wrap your awareness around your entire right foot.

3. Trace your awareness up your lower leg, via your calf, shin, kneecap, back of your knee, thigh and hip. Release and relax your whole right leg.

4. Move your mind toward your right hip, right side of your waist, right shoulder, upper arm, inner elbow, lower arm and wrist. Continue, focusing on the back of your hand, palm, thumb, first finger, second finger, third finger, fourth finger and little finger. Relax your whole right hand and arm.

5. Bring your awareness to your right shoulder, neck, back of your head and forehead. Relax the little frown between the eyebrows; relax your eyes, nose, mouth, tongue. Then bring your awareness to your collarbone. Relax your shoulders, neck and head.

6. Moving down to your chest and stomach, let your stomach relax fully.

7. Repeat on your left-hand side.

8. Relax your entire body, allowing it to be enveloped in your awareness, as if draped in the comforting feeling of being completely safe. You are held, you are safe and you are completely relaxed.

9. Prepare yourself for a deep slumber. Notice the comfort of wherever you're lying or sitting. Notice the quiet and your own slow, steady breathing. Take a few moments to

revel in this cosy, comforting sanctuary before returning to your breath.

10. Come back to your breath while still maintaining that sense of awareness of your whole physical body. See if you can follow the exhale right to the bottom. Notice the pause before the next inhale. You'll see that it's an empty space, where no thought lies. How long does the pause last? Can you hold on to it, or does it slip away before you have time to feel it?

11. Notice the inhalation, starting at the tip of the nose. Bring your awareness to this sensation you can feel at the tip of your nose, right at the start of the inhalation. You might feel a coolness as the air enters through the nose – focus your attention on this feeling.

12. Now for the last minute, just begin again, as though the next inhalation was the first. And with each exhalation, let it be a release. Imagine that you are physically letting go of whatever it is that you need to let go of.

A NOTE ON YOUR PRACTICE

On the face of it, meditation seems simple. Don't worry if your mind wanders off – everyone's does! Just bring your thoughts back when you realize you're thinking about your to-do list again. It may take a while for you to experience the benefits. Be patient – it will come! Practise consistently, and your mind and body will learn that meditation is the signal to relax and get ready for sleep. It's one of those skills that even if you sway out of using it, you can always return.

You could always keep a notebook by the side of your bed to jot down how you've slept, any particularly vivid dreams and whether you feel more refreshed having followed a meditation practice the night before.

My tips for winding down:

- Have a chamomile tea, or anything blended with hops, lemon balm or valerian to help soothe your nervous system before bedtime.

- Cool down: our body temperature decreases as we sleep, unless we are in the throes of menopausal hot flushes! A room that's too hot can prevent us from falling asleep. I often keep the window open all year round, even when it's snowing outside. In the summer I use a cool pad under my feet. I might also keep a cold damp flannel by the side of my bed to cool myself off if I wake in the middle of the night.

- Have an Epsom salt bath: Epsom salts are rich in magnesium. Healthy levels may boost the neurotransmitters responsible for inducing sleep and relaxation, as well as supporting melatonin production. Add them to your bath. They're also an excellent way of hydrating your skin and soothing irritation.

- Use scent: both lavender and chamomile relax our muscles and brain waves. You can find these scents within many night-time body and sleep products. I love a good pillow spray.

- Empty your mind: jot anything whirring around your mind down before switching the light off.

- Read: skip the blue light from a screen – we know this tells the brain it's wake-up time. There is something so much more therapeutic about flicking the pages of a book, folding over the edges when you've had enough.

- Find good noise playlists or sound machines: different noise frequencies have been linked to better quality sleep. White noise (like the hum of a fan) can help mask more disruptive sounds like police sirens and snoring. Pink noise uses deeper, slower sound waves that are particularly soothing and have been shown to promote more stable sleep.[37]

- Don't worry! Lying awake fretting about how little sleep you're getting will only trap you in a vicious cycle. I have been reduced to tears when I'm in an insomnia cycle, a combination of fatigue and utter frustration at myself. Get up, read, do some ironing (repetitive movements can be soporific) – just avoid screens and stick to dim lighting.

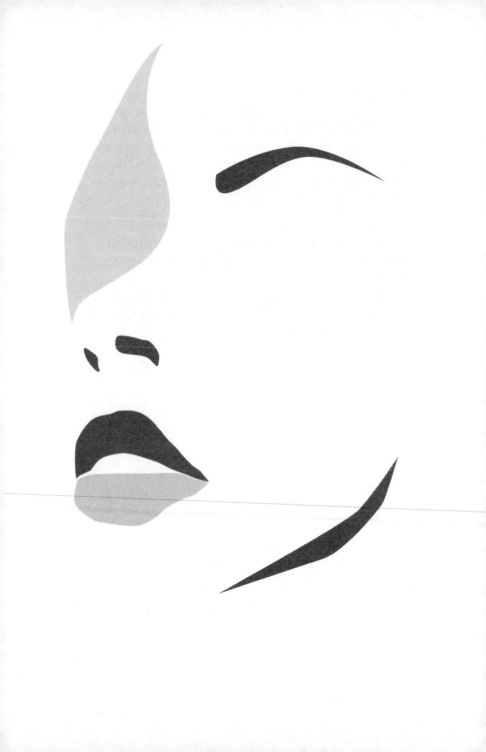

3

Physical Wellness

The Power of Movement

I'm always amazed by how physically active children are. They don't walk; they run, skip, jump, cycle and turn cartwheels with endless energy. So, why does all this stop as we grow older?

During my school years, I was captain of the hockey team, held the record for both the 100m and 200m sprints and spent my weekends horse-riding or helping out with lambing season on my father's rather quirky smallholding. Physical activity wasn't something I planned to do – it was just a part of life. By the time I got to college, and I'd learnt to drive, exercise was no longer a part of my daily routine (although I did spend weekends dancing!). Like most of us, I began to live a more sedentary life.

Many of us spend more than seven hours a day sitting. This means the average person could spend eighteen years of their adult life sitting down![38] Unlike our parents and grandparents, we have desk-based jobs and spend hours commuting, streaming boxsets or scrolling through social media. Such is the impact of this increasingly sedentary lifestyle that sitting has recently been dubbed "the new smoking".[39]

Most of us can't wave a magic wand and leave our desk job, or dedicate half of every day to exercise. But we can build more movement into our day: get up every hour and stretch, jump around

– it all adds up. And don't forget that exercise doesn't just apply to the body. The face and neck are also made up of many muscles and tissues, so maintaining our "facial fitness" with regular massage is a key ingredient to ageing well – from top to toe.

In this chapter, we'll explore how to make small changes that, day by day, add up to a big difference. By moving well and often, we'll begin to age better too.

Rebounding

Let's face it; not all of us find a form of exercise they are good at and actually enjoy. With rebounding, you simply bounce on a mini-trampoline – nobody says we have to stop having fun with our physical movement as we get older! As you rise, you experience a feeling of weightless; as your feet press into the trampoline, your body can experience up to 4Gs of gravitational force, bringing a multitude of benefits – and it's also so much fun!

How to get started:

1. Practice controlling your acceleration and deceleration by using the power in your legs and engaging your core.

2. When you've got the hang of it, you can add in jumping jacks, twists (your body and legs go one way; your arms go the other) and even using a skipping rope as you bounce.

3. Start with 3 minutes at a time, then aim to build up to at least 15 minutes, three times a week.

Exercise and Brain Chemistry

We're all familiar with the idea that exercise can help us maintain weight and keep our hearts healthy. Physical activity burns calories, increases muscle tone and keeps our heart functioning well – all great reasons to make exercise a non-negotiable habit. Yet the benefits of exercise run deeper – and it all starts with our brain chemistry.

When we exercise, our body releases endorphins – feel-good neurotransmitters made in the brain. Endorphins are the reason people talk about experiencing a "runner's high".[40] Regular exercise can reduce stress hormones (cortisol and adrenalin), which, as we saw in Chapter 1, contribute to collagen breakdown and skin ageing.

Even better, physical activity triggers the release of serotonin (the happy hormone), norepinephrine (low levels of which are associated with depression) and dopamine – a key regulator for both your mood and sleep/wake cycle.[41]

Working Out to Get Your Glow

When we talk about someone having a healthy glow, it's often because they've been for a brisk walk in cold air, returned from a run or have emerged from a yoga class. They look rosy-cheeked, with plump, glowing skin – all the immediate benefits from exercising.

It doesn't stop there. As our body temperature rises, the eccrine glands (found mainly in your armpits and groin) produce sweat. As this moisture (a mix of water, salt and fat) evaporates from our skin, it lowers our body temperature and cools us down. It also brings important skin benefits, and can help remove dirt, oil, pollution and dead skin cells from our pores, reducing breakouts and acne flare-ups. Sweat is also the source of an antimicrobial peptide called dermcidin which helps protect against infection from harmful germs, behaving like a natural antibiotic.[42]

Like sweat, blood flow increases when we exercise, as our heart rate increases to pump blood to muscles around the body. The increase in blood circulation helps remove waste products and deliver a fresh supply of oxygen and nutrients to skin cells. As lymphatic drainage improves, fluid trapped in tissues is returned to the body's central circulation system, reducing puffiness – particularly around the eyes.[43] So, even after just a single workout, our skin recovers its healthy glow.

Exercise and DNA

Beyond the healthy glow and feel-good factor, exercise creates changes within the skin at a cellular level. As we know from Chapter 1, telomeres are small protective tips that sit at the end of DNA strands. Over time, these telomeres get shorter, accelerating the ageing process. Scientists have found that regular exercise can increase the length of our telomeres, helping to stave off ageing.[44]

Exercise and cell energy

Exercise has the power to do things that even modern medicine hasn't yet been able to replicate. Take mitochondria, which act like an engine within almost every cell in our body Mitochondria make a chemical called ATP (adenosine 5'-triphosphate): a substance involved in repairing damage and making essential skin components like collagen and hyaluronic acid. Over time, the mitochondria start to produce less ATP (energy) and our skin appears older. What's astonishing is that while no medication has been able to restore the youthful function of mitochondria, one study showed that exercise could reverse these changes that occur within our muscles as we age.[45] What's more, those who exercise regularly may have a thicker dermis (the second layer within the skin)[46] and develop fewer lines and wrinkles. When we come onto facial treatments in Chapter 6, we'll see that those such as microcurrent and LED therapy also have the ability to stimulate ATP.

Exercise and the "youth switch"

Longevity science is a fascinating study in extending our lifespans. One important discovery is AMPK (adenosine monophosphate-activated protein kinase): an enzyme that regulates cell energy. It's often referred to as the body's "youth switch" for its ability to decrease many symptoms associated with chronic conditions and ageing[47] by turning on youthful cell function.[48] Unsurprisingly, AMPK declines as we age. Exercise has been linked with increased AMPK activity,[49] helping our body behave younger than our years!

A NOTE ON
EXERCISE AND INFLAMMATORY SKIN CONDITIONS

It's worth mentioning that exercise can be a challenge for those suffering from conditions such as eczema and rosacea. Sodium within sweat, coupled with the loss of moisture, can increase skin dryness and irritation.[50] Likewise, the rise in body temperature and increased blood supply can be challenging for those with rosacea conditions.

That said, the long list of benefits that come with exercise means you shouldn't be put off from finding a workout you enjoy. If your skin is suffering, exercise somewhere where there's air conditioning and avoid hot yoga or running in direct sunlight. Stay hydrated and wear clothes that aren't too tight or rub against your skin. Shorter bursts and/or lower-intensity workouts can also be a huge help. Don't forget to use products that help repair your skin barrier and protect you from UV light (particularly if you're exercising outside).

The Simplicity of Walking

I've tried all kinds of weird and wonderful ways to work out. But let's not forget how simple walking is. Walking is free (fancy leggings optional), accessible and one of the most underrated ways of staying active.

Walking can help improve our endurance, circulation, posture and cardiac health while preventing weight gain and even lowering our risk of cancer, heart diseases and other chronic illnesses.[51] In comparing moderate-intensity walking with vigorous running, researchers found that both result in a similarly reduced risk of high blood pressure, high cholesterol and diabetes.[52]

Gentle walking after meals can improve digestion by stimulating the stomach and intestines, helping food pass through more quickly. It may even help alleviate the symptoms of irritable bowel syndrome (IBS)[53] and regulate blood sugar levels.

As for our mental wellbeing, researchers at Stanford University found that walking increased people's creative output by up to 60 per cent.[54] Others have noted that just twelve minutes walking a day can lead to increased happiness and self-confidence.[55]

If the science isn't compelling enough, just thinking about my favourite places to walk near my home in the countryside makes me a believer in the power of walking. Even twenty minutes is enough to help lower my stress levels, refresh my brain and allow my thoughts to flow more freely. For me, walking is like medicine – partly because it invites us into the great outdoors.

What's All the Fuss About Vitamin N?

When I was a child, getting a blast of fresh air or "blowing away the cobwebs" was seen as the remedy for all kinds of physical ailments and low mood blues. In the last few years, we've come to link spending time outdoors with getting our fix of vitamin D. An essential nutrient for bone health, vitamin D is made by our skin when exposed to sunlight, yet 40 per cent of Europeans are now deficient in it.[56]

So, what's vitamin N – and how is it related to health and ageing? The Global Wellness Summit recently reported that a growing number of doctors have begun "prescribing nature" to patients living predominantly indoors within urban environments. It makes sense, given that Dutch researchers found a lower incidence of fifteen diseases, including depression, anxiety, heart disease, diabetes, asthma and migraines, in people who lived within about a half-mile of green space.[57]

Experts now recommend that we all get a thirty-minute dose of vitamin N (nature) each day.[58] If we want to stay healthy and age better, it's time to swap the sofa sessions for more exercise, preferably outside with Mother Nature.

Yoga for Glowing Skin

I'm aware of the clichés that come with being a yoga bunny. Finding myself juggling work and the demands of a young family, my stress levels were through the roof, so I took myself off to yoga as a way to get some time for myself, physically and emotionally. The tools I've gained from yoga – for maintaining both physical and emotional wellbeing – are life-changing. You don't need to practise daily but once you learn the basics, yoga stays with you for life.

It's well known that yoga lowers stress levels, helping us cope with challenging situations more effectively. By reducing the body's stress response, we can lower our risk of skin flare-ups. Yoga can also help redress what we referred to in Chapter 1 as "skin-flammageing". A study by the National Institutes of Health found that regular yogis had a 22 per cent reduction in inflammation indicators, which could otherwise contribute to collagen breakdown and cellular ageing.[59] Yoga also supports the lymphatic system – the body's natural detoxification process – making for clearer, more vibrant skin.

Yoga benefits us in a multitude of ways. Yet when it comes to our skin, inversions – or any pose that involves raising your heart above your head (something as simple as a forward bend with your head down) – are particularly useful in bringing blood flow to our face. Increased blood flow delivers oxygen and vital nutrients to our skin cells, helping them to function more effectively, accelerate repair, promote elasticity and lessen the appearance of scars.[60] Apart from anything else, yoga makes me happier. I firmly believe that happiness is an essential ingredient for living well and staying youthful.

———————————

Hormones and Skin Changes

Hormones are part of the endocrine system, and they play a vital role in how our skin looks, feels and ages. Just as our stress hormones (cortisol and adrenalin) affect our skin, the major reproductive hormones (oestrogen, progesterone and testosterone) determine its health and appearance.

Our hormones change on a weekly, monthly and yearly basis as we move from our teenage years, through pregnancy, perimenopause and menopause. By understanding how your hormones behave throughout your cycle and as you age, you can get to know your skin better and treat it accordingly.

Oestrogen: the female hormone that makes our skin appear plump, dewy and youthful. It declines as we age.

Testosterone: the male hormone that results in oilier, thicker skin and stimulates collagen production. In women, it helps repair tissues, muscle and bone function and maintains metabolic health.

Progesterone: a female hormone that is also present in men. It plays a key role during pregnancy and stimulates sebum production.

Your skin during your cycle

During your period (follicular phase): your menstrual cycle begins on the first day of your period and ends when your next period starts. During your period, low levels of oestrogen can mean your skin feel a little dry. Conversely, in some people, the drop in these hormones can also trigger sebum production and inflammation, leading to acne.

After your period (proliferative phase): as oestrogen levels rise, promoting collagen production, your skin appears stronger and plumper. Spots should start clearing up.

Mid-cycle ovulation: oestrogen levels peak just before ovulation. Some people find that their skin takes on a natural glow at this point in their cycle.

After ovulation (luteal phase): as your body releases progesterone and stimulates sebum production, you may find your pores become clogged, and your skin becomes more prone to spots.

Before your period (secretory phase): increased levels of progesterone can lead to water retention and your face may appear puffier than usual.

Oestrogen and Ageing

In the early 1920s, researchers Edgar Allen and Edward Adelbert Doisy conducted experiments that led to the discovery of oestrogen and the role it plays in female reproduction.[61] Since then, scientists have discovered that oestrogen has many more protective functions, affecting our bones, brain, colon and vascular system, to name a few.[62] Oestrogen also impacts how our skin looks and ages.

Throughout our lifetime, oestrogen levels tend to peak around our late twenties, decreasing by 50 per cent at the age of fifty and dropping off during menopause.[63] Oestrogen promotes skin elasticity, hydration and thickness, giving us a plump, dewy glow.[64] As oestrogen levels decline, collagen production within both our skin and bones slows. Our skin loses its tone, plumpness and structure, so wrinkles appear.

Falling oestrogen levels and menopause are, of course, a natural part of life – and are certainly not things we should fear. If it's something you decide is right for you, hormone replacement therapy (HRT) could increase skin hydration, elasticity and thickness. It can also improve the quality of collagen within our skin and reduce the appearance of wrinkles.[65]

I, like my mother, started an early menopause. The first symptoms emerged around the age of forty-one, but I was forty-five before I sought medical help. From being on HRT for three months the improvement in so many aspects of my health was huge: it helped with my mental health, my physical aches and pains and absolutely increased skin springiness! HRT was not something I ever thought I would consider, as I try where possible to follow a more holistic method. I also take supplements to support this area of my health, but this really has been life-changing for the better.

Whether you decide to go down that route or not, staying physically active and maintaining healthy, radiant skin – and the confidence that comes with it – is possible at any age. The tips at the end of this chapter, along with the four-week plan, will help you and your skin stay youthful for longer.

Your Physical Wellness Toolkit

Whether you're getting back into exercise, looking for some new ideas or simply want to invest more time in taking care of your body, here are some practices I rely on to keep me feeling good and looking youthful.

Dry body brushing

I learnt about dry body brushing as a young spa therapist, but it makes for the ideal home beauty ritual. It dates back to Ayurvedic cultures, as well as in Ancient Egyptian and Chinese medicine. Dry body brushing involves buffing dry skin with a brush, leaving your skin softer and smoother. Sloughing off dead cells also allows any body products you apply afterwards to penetrate deeper and work more effectively.

Beyond the surface-level benefits, dry body brushing helps keep our body functioning well from the inside out. Helping to boost circulation and increase blood flow, it also stimulates lymphatic drainage and detoxification. I often do it in the morning before showering, two to three times a week. Be careful to avoid any areas with broken skin, inflammation, eczema or dermatitis.

1. Choose a brush with soft but firm bristles and a long handle so that you can reach your back.

2. On dry skin, start at your feet and use long, circular sweeping motions with medium pressure. Work upward, moving in the direction of your heart. From feet to knee, then knee to groin. You can be firmer on your thighs and bottom.

3. When you reach your chest, use downward strokes from beneath your jaw toward your heart to encourage lymphatic drainage. You will want to be gentler on your décolletage.

4. Sweep up from hands to elbows then elbow to armpit.

5. Shower and follow with a hydrating body moisturizer.

Cold bathing

Like dry body brushing, this is something I covered in my early training as a spa therapist for the body and for the face. But really, cold bathing is embedded in my family's history.

My father vividly remembers being woken up at 4am every morning by the sound of his father taking a cold shower before heading off to work in the Birmingham fish markets. Cold bathing is now part of my father's life. He's even developed his own outdoor bath: a converted cattle trough, enamelled inside with a beer cooler attached to maintain a low water temperature.

Cold Water Immersion (CWI) has recently attracted media attention thanks to proponents such as Wim Hof a.k.a. "The Iceman", who holds the Guinness World Record for swimming under ice. However, it's been around for centuries; the Ancient Greeks experimented with variously hot and cold pools.

Cold bathing may sound horrendous (particularly on a winter's morning!) but the science speaks volumes. Cold water stimulates the lymphatic system and triggers the immune system's white blood cells, helping the body flush out toxins and fight infection. Like exercise, cold water also increases blood flow and improves cardiovascular circulation to keep our heart healthy and supply our organs with vital nutrients.[66]

Cold bathing can increase our metabolic rate by up to 16 per cent, thereby helping us lose weight.[67] One study even found that regular cold showers could help alleviate the symptoms of depression and lift mood.[68] Get through the first few seconds, and you're likely to feel more energized and sharper mentally as you prepare to face your day.

Let's not forget that cold water brings a host of immediate benefits to our skin – from reducing under-eye puffiness to minimizng the appearance of pores, stimulating nutrient-rich blood flow to our cells and relieving tension. While hot water can strip the skin of its natural oils, aggravating inflammatory conditions, cold water can calm and soothe while also bringing a natural healthy glow to all complexions. All skin types and conditions will benefit from cold therapy.

My tips for cold bathing:

- You can fill a bath with cold water (my personal preference); however you might find it easier and more practical to take a cold shower.

- Start slow: you can begin and end your shower with a cold blast of water and/or gradually lower the temperature bit by bit each day.

- Breathe! This is not going to be pleasant to start with, but slowing your breathing rate will help you control your body's response to the cold and is a key component to the process (you will find you begin to crave the cold feeling if you make it a regular practice!). Slow, full, deep breaths.

- Be consistent: you could start with just fifteen to thirty seconds and build up to two to five minutes. Try and have a cold shower every day to get the health benefits. If it's a cold bath, once you are in and under the water it actually feels quite comfortable!

- Be aware your body might actually feel warm when you immediately get out. However, make sure you wrap up warm afterward to help the body restore its temperature balance. You might want a warm shower directly following the cold bathing; some days I do and others not.

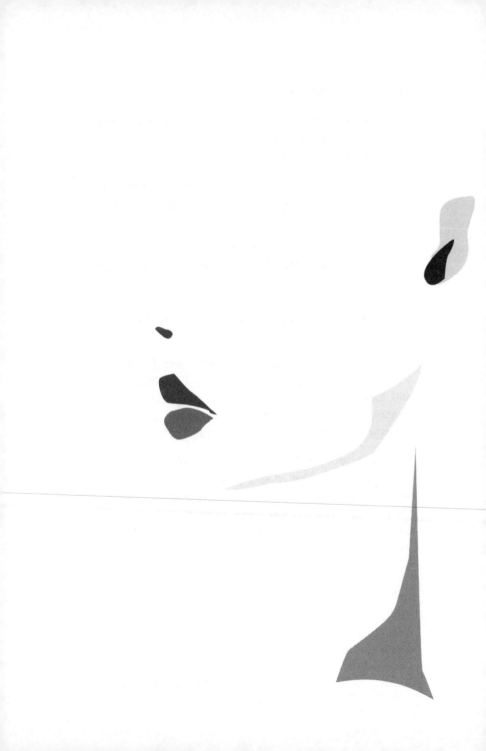

4

External Stress

From the Outside In

Ageing is the one thing in life that connects us globally. It's a total gift to be able to develop lines that mark the passage of time and tell our life story on our faces. Most of us would like to age in the best possible way – not everyone wants to be wrinkle-free; most of us want to look glowing and good for our age. There are two key factors we need to take into consideration: the genes we are born with and the life we lead.

As we've seen, many factors affect ageing. Some of these factors are within our power to influence, others less so. To distinguish between the two, it can be helpful to think about "intrinsic" and "extrinsic" ageing.

Intrinsic ageing is what we're born with – and largely beyond our control. Our genetics play a huge role in determining the rate at which our collagen production declines, our eyes become more hooded and we begin to develop lines and wrinkles. The best marker for intrinsic ageing is your parents, and the older generations within your family. It's a cliché but the vast majority of us do find ourselves looking more and more like our parents as we age.

Extrinsic ageing is more about how external lifestyle factors affect us. Think about the climate you live in, the amount of exposure you have to the sun, your stress levels, your diet and whether you smoke or take medication or the contraceptive pill. As these are things you can influence, they will be our focus for this chapter.

Pollution and Ageing – the New Skin Threat?

Airborne pollution is: "the contamination of outdoor and indoor environments by any chemical, physical or biological agent that modifies the natural characteristics of the atmosphere".[69]

According to the World Health Organization (WHO), air pollution kills around seven million people worldwide every year, as a result of increased rates of stroke, heart disease, chronic obstructive pulmonary disease, lung cancer and acute respiratory infections. And it's not just people who live in notoriously smoggy cities. Nine out of ten of us breathe air that exceeds WHO guideline limits of pollutants.[70]

Outdoor pollutants

The primary outdoor air pollutants are nitrogen dioxide, sulphur dioxide, carbon monoxide, particulate matter (microscopic particles of dust and dirt in the air) and heavy metals. Many pollutants become more toxic when they interact with the sun's UV light.[71]

Indoor pollutants

As most of us spend around 90 per cent of our lives inside[72] – at work or in our homes – indoor pollution also has a hugely significant impact on our overall health. Exposure to indoor pollutants comes via cigarette smoke, heating, cooking, poor ventilation and damp, as well as chemicals within household cleaning products, plastics and some building materials.

Indirect exposure, which occurs when we inhale and ingest pollutants, also negatively impacts both the superficial and deep levels of our skin, increasing cell death and decreasing cell proliferation.[73] So, pollution is showing up on our skin day-to-day – and accelerating how fast we age.

Pollution and inflammation

We already know that inflammation plays a vital role in the ageing process. Pollution can activate our inflammatory processes, thereby exacerbating conditions like eczema and dermatitis. Living in a highly polluted environment is also linked to atopy – a genetic tendency toward having a heightened response to common allergens.[74] This increased sensitivity shows up on our skin as redness and flaking and is why we often hear about atopic eczema.

Pollution and skin ageing

Free radicals are oxygen-containing molecules with an uneven number of electrons that can trigger chemical reactions called "oxidation" within the body. We need some free radicals to fight bacteria. But when the number of free radicals outweighs the number of antioxidants (substances that inhibit oxidation), we suffer oxidative stress. This stress causes our cells to become damaged.

Pollution both lowers the level of antioxidants (such as vitamins C and E) within our skin, and induces oxidation of vital skin components such as squalene (a lipid that keeps skin smooth and hydrated). As a result, pollution has been linked to an increase in pigmented age spots, deep nasolabial folds (wrinkles that run from the nose to the corners of the mouth) and skin sagging. Exposure to UV light seems to have a double whammy effect: smokers who experience higher exposure to sunlight have been found to have more wrinkles on their forehead and cheeks.[75]

Pollution and acne

As well as triggering inflammation-causing acne, pollution exposure is also associated with an increase in the skin's sebum (oil) production and related flare-ups.[76]

Pollution and the skin microbiome

In Chapter 1, we looked at how stress can negatively impact the skin microbiome – or the eco-system of living organisms that are unique to every one of us. Just as stress can disturb the delicate balance of the skin microbiome, pollution can alter its composition. This imbalance triggers a wide variety of reactions that accelerate ageing.[77]

Chemicals are everywhere and, in many cases, exposure is beyond our control, so it's important not to feel overwhelmed. However, there are things we can do to reduce external stressors on our health and skin – like deciding not to smoke (this includes e-cigarettes). We can also rethink our household cleaning products. If you're commuting into a city, look into different travel routes – is there a journey that would avoid the busiest roads, or even bypass peak traffic times?

As far as quick wins go, the best thing you can do after a day at work is to cleanse your face as soon as you get home, rather than waiting until bedtime. If your skin is really suffering from the effects of pollution, you could travel make-up free in the morning, cleanse when you reach the office – then put your face on. This way, the pollution from your morning commute won't sit on the surface of your skin all day.

———

Let's Talk Central Heating

Like most people, I rely on central heating to keep warm. The problem with this is that like many people, I could go from home to an office and back home again, spending the vast majority of the winter season in an environment that's totally unsuitable for my skin.

A study in America found that eczema rates were lower in parts of the country where people have increased sun exposure and live in a more humid environment.[78] By contrast, anyone who suffers from eczema or dermatitis will know that flare-ups, itching and flaking tend to be worse in winter.

Central heating (just like air conditioning) reduces the moisture levels in the air. The fall in humidity draws moisture from our skin, causing it to become dry and tight. It might even become rough in texture, scaly and prone to flaking. Low humidity also compromises our skin's barrier function, so it becomes more reactive to irritants and allergens.[79]

It's not only having the thermostat turned up to tropical that impacts our skin. The sharp contrast in temperature as we move from indoors to outdoors also causes our blood vessels to dilate, making redness, acne and rosacea appear worse. Even the most robust skins can suffer from dryness, with lines and wrinkles becoming more visible in the colder months. Don't forget, this is also the time of the year when many of us are also lacking in vitamin D.

The next step to protecting your skin against external stress is choosing the right products that support – rather than irritate – your skin barrier. A strong skin barrier means healthier skin that stays youthful for longer.

Barrier Function for Youthful Skin

Scientists have known about the skin barrier for decades. More recently, a whole host of skincare products claiming to strengthen its function have landed in stores and online.

Nevertheless, the skin barrier is often misunderstood. Because of its name ("barrier") and the fact that it literally forms the boundary between our internal and external environments, people often mistakenly assume that barrier function relates to the surface level of our skin only. Actually, the skin barrier plays an essential role in overall skin health and ageing.

The skin is the largest organ in the body. The outer layer of skin (or epidermis) is barely thicker than a piece of paper, yet it provides vital defence against water loss, UV exposure and infection. Without it, we would die.

The skin barrier begins at the stratum corneum – the very outermost layer of the epidermis – which is structured like a brick wall. Cells called corneocytes are the "bricks" and lipids are the "mortar" that keeps it all together.

Along with the skin microbiome, the acid mantle (a film of water and oil) covers the surface and contributes to healthy barrier function. When our acid mantle is intact, the natural acidity helps maintain the low pH of the skin. In doing so, it inhibits the growth of harmful bacteria, prevents toxins from being absorbed into the skin, acts as a lubricant and limits trans-epidermal water loss that leads to dryness.

So, one of the skin's primary roles is to form barrier defence systems. Yet, when one system is damaged, it triggers a domino effect that impacts other cells within the body.[80] So the function of the skin barrier is much more than just skin deep.

Contrary to many skincare brand claims, it's not necessarily the deeper layers that need all the focus. Rather, it's the stratum corneum and skin barrier that needs support if we're to maintain healthy, youthful-looking skin.[81] As the skin barrier can influence regeneration within the deeper layers of the skin, it makes sense that it should be one of our first considerations when building our skincare routine.

A NOTE ON IRRITANTS

As an aesthetician, I've been lucky enough to have tried and tested many different products over the years. I've lost count of the number of times I've been asked "What's the best anti-wrinkle cream?" (sorry, there's no silver bullet), or "How can I eliminate dark circles?" (no quick fixes here either!). Perhaps surprisingly, the most important thing I've learnt from decades of testing products is the effect they have on my skin barrier.

Ever since I was a child, my skin has been prone to sensitivity. If I use the wrong type of product – or continue using certain formulations for too long – my skin barrier will always let me know that it's unhappy. I quickly retreat to the safety of my regular clinical and cosmeceutical (a cross between a cosmetic and pharmaceutical formula) products.

A good skincare plan is like a good diet: it has plenty of nutritious ingredients – and far fewer damaging ones. Before we start building your skincare routine with the right balance of product types and ingredients, it's worth thinking about what you might need to reduce or cut out entirely.

In my experience of seeing thousands of clients, products that disrupt the skin barrier are often behind a long list of skin issues. Here are some important ones to watch out for. Please keep in mind it's all about everything in balance!

Exfoliating acids

You might see these labelled as AHAs (alpha-hydroxy acids), BHAs (beta-hydroxy acids) or PHAs (polyhydroxy acids). They bring a wealth of different skin benefits – from speeding up cell turnover, reducing lines and restoring plumpness to fighting acne – and are an important part of your routine. I love a good acid! However, acid junkies be warned: use too many and your skin can become red, irritated, photosensitive and prone to pigmentation and breakouts.

Overuse can also stop your skin from producing healthy new cells, damage the acid mantle of your skin barrier and result in acne.

Surfactants

The name surfactants refers to the fact that they are "surface active agents", often used in cleansers (as well as shampoos and body washes) to create a foam, but are often very drying on the skin and can cause sensitivity. One example of as surfactant is sodium lauryl sulphate.

Emulsifiers

Emulsifiers (such as benzalkonium chloride, behentrimonium methosulphate, cetearyl alcohol, stearic acid, glyceryl stearate and ceteareth-20) are agents within skin creams that allow water and oils to mix (just as you might add mustard to bind your salad dressing). Although some research suggests that they can help enhance the absorption of skincare ingredients,[82] they may modify the lipid (mortar) layers within the stratum corneum and compromise the skin barrier, causing irritation. Emulsifiers are often described as having a "wash-out" effect, as they trigger an increase in the loss of protective skin substances, thereby washing out the good.[83]

Synthetic preservatives

Just as the name suggests, preservatives (such as parabens and formaldehyde-releasing ingredients and diazolidinyl urea) are there to preserve your skin products by preventing them from becoming contaminated by harmful bacteria. They're necessary (especially in jar-based creams which we dip our fingers in and out of), and not all preservatives are bad. Ones to watch out for include parabens and formaldehyde-releasing ingredients like diazolidinyl urea, which have been linked to hormonal disruption and may even be carcinogenic. Other preservatives that are thought to be safer include benzyl alcohol, citric acid, potassium sorbate and sorbic acid.

Fragrance

Of course, skincare isn't just about what it *does* — it's about how it makes you feel. Yet, while a beautifully scented moisturizer might feel like a treat, fragrances (such as eugenol, geraniol, citronellol, farnesol and cinnamyl alcohol) can rob your skin of skin barrier-repairing ingredients, making it more sensitive. Even if you're not someone who typically sees a reaction to fragranced products, they could be causing harm deep down (much like UV damage). Over time, this "invisible" damage can accumulate and compromise your skin's health and radiance. If you have eczema or sensitivity, avoid fragrance like the plague.

Drying alcohols

Drying alcohols (such as denatured alcohol) can give skincare products a lovely, weightless texture — and may even help ingredients such as retinol vitamin C penetrate more effectively. The problem is, certain types of alcohol do this by breaking down the skin barrier, destroying its crucial line of defence. There are, however, other types of alcohol, known as "fatty alcohols" (cetyl, stearyl and cetearyl alcohol) that are non-irritating.[84]

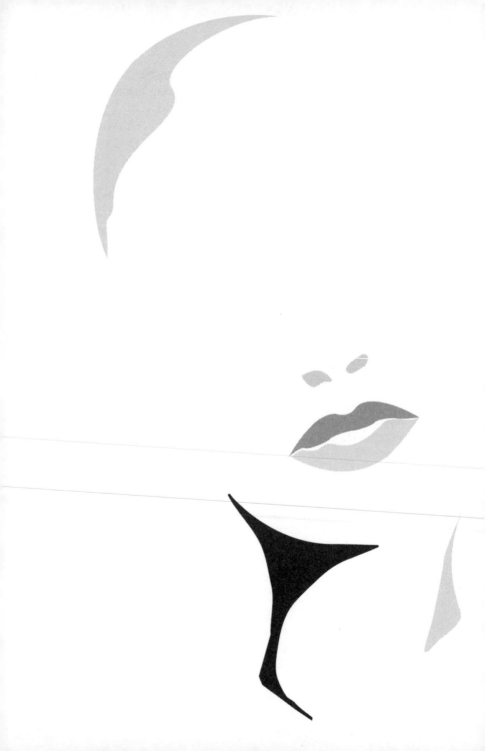

5

Eating Well to Age Better

The Missing Link to Glowing Skin

I could write a whole book on the topic of food, gut health and skin. However, I've done my best to cover the points I hope you'll find most helpful in this chapter.

I was raised in a foodie family. My grandmother (a devout vegetarian who suffered from Coeliac disease) kept bees and made all her food from scratch. There was always some gluten-free bread or a nut loaf baking in the oven when I went to stay.

Not uncommonly, I developed an eating disorder in my teens. Later, suffering a whole host of digestive issues, I was told I may have IBS (Irritable Bowel Syndrome). I'm sure some of my gut issues were connected to stress. I underwent every test under the sun – had tiny cameras inserted at both ends – and still, doctors and consultants couldn't pinpoint the cause of the sudden flare-ups that kept me in bed for days. Fed up with the pain, the exhaustion and the seemingly eternal brain fog, I went gluten-free for three years, I took allergy tests, went on juice diets, stuck to eating raw food and tried all kinds of hokey pokey, desperate to feel good again. For twenty years, I found nothing that worked. I know from my work in my skin clinic these types of stories are not uncommon.

At long last, I was diagnosed with a form of IBD (Inflammatory Bowel Disease, microscopic colitis) and learnt to recognize foods and lifestyle factors that trigger my symptoms – and how to manage things better.

It's perhaps because of my digestive history that I'm such a believer in the power of nutrition. While I'm not a qualified nutritionist, I have more than enough anecdotal evidence from my clients to know that supporting digestion, reducing internal inflammation and fuelling our bodies the right way all helps keep our skin youthful and our health on track. My digestive problems didn't make my skin break out, but did cause sensitivity and many other issues throughout my body. Digestive issues manifest themselves in very different ways from person to person.

Topically, we can use the power of touch, technology and products. All of these will benefit your skin. However, don't underestimate the power of food and supplements. Together, they're the missing link to getting glowing skin for life.

Amazingly, with 40 trillion bacterial cells and 30 trillion human cells, we're actually more bacteria than human! There are up to 1,000 species of bacteria in our intestines, and together, they can weigh 1–2kg – roughly the same weight as our brain. So, our microbiome (the delicate eco-system of micro-organisms within our gut) is as important as an organ and is closely linked with our immune system, brain, heart health and risk of serious illness.

Beyond our physical health, the gut also plays a crucial role in our mental wellbeing. In fact, research suggests that our mind and gut have a symbiotic relationship: by altering the balance of bacteria within our gut, we can potentially become happier and bolder. Likewise, even moderate stress can negatively impact the healthy balance of our microbiome. Incredibly, gut bacteria are thought to manufacture around 95 per cent of the body's serotonin – or "happy hormone".

This is why our gut is often referred to as our second brain – and why the saying "gut feeling" may be much more than an old wives' tale!

Science is evolving all the time, but the link between mental health conditions (stress and anxiety), digestive disorders (Crohn's disease, IBS, etc.) and our skin is becoming increasingly apparent. So, if we want to age well, it's essential that we pay attention to our gut.

Feeding Your Skin Cells to Age Well

As our largest organ, the skin acts as a mirror for what's going on inside our body. Eat well, and our skin looks healthy, plump and glowing. When too much sugar, dairy, gluten, processed foods and alcohol creep in, our skin can often send us a message in the form of breakouts, dry patches, eczema, inflammation and redness. Our complexion becomes dull and lacklustre with more and more tell-tale lines.

Just as we looked at the key components within your skincare plan, balancing your diet and taking the right supplements can be a game-changer if you want your skin to stay healthy and vibrant for longer.

Macro and micronutrients

Let's start with the building blocks of good nutrition. Macronutrients are carbohydrates, proteins and lipids that we require in large amounts to maintain our health. Micronutrients include minerals like sodium, copper and zinc, along with vitamins such as A, B, C, D and E. They are referred to as "micro" because the body only needs them in trace amounts. I love that the World Health Organization (WHO) refers to micronutrients as the "magic wands" that enable the body to produce enzymes, hormones and other substances essential for proper growth and development.[85] Macro and micronutrients work together to maintain the barrier function and integrity of our skin. On the next page I explore these nutrients in more detail.

Carbohydrates

As the fuel for our body's engine, carbohydrates produce glucose to support cellular activities, including the production of fibroblasts (which synthesize collagen) and secretion of hormones and growth factors. They are far too often given a bad reputation, but they play a key part in a balanced diet.

Protein

As an essential component of immune system cells, protein activates macrophages: specialized cells involved in detecting and destroying harmful bacteria. Protein is also needed for wound healing.

Essential amino acids

Of the many amino acids, some are referred to as essential because the body is unable to produce them by itself. This means we must get them from our diet. As the building blocks of peptides and protein (collagen being a key protein for skin) they perform a variety of skin-essential roles – helping to maintain hydration levels, support the immune system, protect against free radical damage and reduce the signs of ageing.

Examples include arginine (in chicken, pumpkin seeds and spirulina), which deposits collagen and reduces damage; histidine (in dairy, poultry, nuts and seeds), which soothes the skin and has antioxidant properties; methionine (in eggs, grains and seeds), which defends against harmful substances; and lysine (in meat, poultry, sardines, soy beans) to strengthen the skin's surface. Proline (in egg whites, dairy, cabbage and asparagus), leucine (in salmon, chickpeas and brown rice) and glycine (in meat, fish, dairy, kidney beans and lentils) can help reduce the depth of lines and wrinkles.[86]

Peptides

Peptides are short strings of amino acids found naturally within our skin and in food sources. As the foundation for collagen and elastin fibres, they play a significant part in keeping our skin healthy and youthful.

Essential Fatty Acids (EFAs)

Like amino acids, most are "essential", so must be obtained from food and supplements. The most important ones to mention here are Omegas 3 and 6, as these are the only ones that are literally essential. They regulate the inflammatory response, protect against sun damage, maintain cell membrane health, strengthen barrier function and help keep our skin hydrated, plump and youthful.

Lipids

Lipids are fats. They are a vital component of cell membranes that helps regulate cellular inflammation and metabolism and plays a role in blood flow and clotting. Specialized lipids are required for the development of the skin's stratum corneum (outermost layer).[87]

Minerals

We need copper to support the repair of collagen and tissues. Zinc is involved in collagen synthesis; manganese is needed for tissue regeneration.

Antioxidants

Exposure to UV light, pollution, chemicals and stress is an inevitable part of life. Getting a good supply of antioxidants from vitamins helps neutralize the effects of free radicals that accelerate ageing.

Vitamin A: supports our immune system, promotes collagen production and guards against the effects of inflammation (although too much can be harmful).

B vitamins: this refers to a group of vitamins, which have slightly different functions. Vitamins B2 and B5 can help reduce skin oiliness, B2 (riboflavin) is essential for healthy cell growth, B3 (niacin) helps maintain barrier function to relieve eczema and rosacea. A very pale complexion can be a sign of vitamin B deficiency, as can cracks at the side of your mouth.

Vitamin C: found within both the epidermal and dermal layers of our skin. It declines with age and exposure to external stressors, yet both oral supplementation and topical application of vitamin C products have been found to increase levels within the skin.[88] As one of the most important skin vitamins, it supports collagen production and cell regeneration, boosts our resistance to infection and promotes iron absorption.

Vitamin D: this vitamin has a complex relationship with the skin. We know that too much UV radiation can damage our skin, causing premature ageing and cancer. Conversely, cells within the epidermis are responsible for making vitamin D when exposed to sunlight. Vitamin D is involved in the protection of skin, the destruction of free radicals and the growth, repair and metabolism of our cells.[89] As it's also responsible for maintaining bone strength, we need it to keep our bodies strong and youthful.

Vitamin E: when we talk about vitamin E, we're referring to a group of molecules that are delivered to the upper layers of skin via sebum.[90] As an important antioxidant, it helps protect against free radical damage by absorbing radiation from UV light.[91]

Flavonoids

These are molecules found in fruit and vegetables (often referred to as "phytonutrients") that act like a natural sunscreen, helping to defend the skin against UV ageing while repairing DNA damage. They can also protect our blood vessels and reduce the likelihood of us developing broken capillaries (spider veins) near the skin surface.[92]

Water

We've probably all been told to drink more water at some point or other. Not only does water make up 64 per cent of our skin,[93] but it's also involved in almost every bodily function. As a major component of blood, it helps dissolve vitamins, minerals, glucose and amino acids before transporting them to our cells. So, if we want to glow, we need to drink water – and lots of it. There are a number of foods which also have a high water content, so a huge yes to drinking water, but also consider *eating* water. Think cucumbers, watermelons, lettuce.

Why is Wound Healing so Important?

When we hear about "wound healing", our mind often jumps to cuts or serious injuries. Actually, in the beauty world, it's inherently linked to skin ageing and many of the treatments carried out in clinics such as micro-needling, derma-pen, fractional radio frequency and some lasers use this wound healing response to stimulate new collagen production and create a more youthful complexion and reduce the appearance of wrinkles and scars.

Researchers began documenting this process as early as World War I when they noticed that older soldiers appeared to heal slower than younger ones.[94] So, wound healing simply refers to our body's ability to replace destroyed or damaged tissue with healthy new tissue. It's one of the most complex processes to occur within the human body and involves communication and coordination between the skin and immune cells. This communication gets disrupted as we age. This is why you may have noticed that as you've gotten older, cuts, bruises and scars take longer to fade.

Beneath the skin surface, our body's ability to resist and repair damage also slows as we age. The network of collagen within our skin becomes "stiffer", delaying the inflammatory response needed to repair damage. As our fibroblasts lose the ability to function effectively, we begin to lose the youthful plumpness of our skin.[95]

The nutrients we get from our food and supplements – as well as topical products – can support this wound healing process, helping our skin remain resilient to the effects of ageing.

Digestive Disorders and Skin Health

As someone who suffered from digestive disorders this subject couldn't be closer to my heart. As I know all too well, having long-term digestive issues won't just leave you miserable, exhausted and in pain – it'll compromise the health and vitality of your skin too.

As we discovered in previous chapters, the health of our skin is intricately bound with the balance and diversity of bacteria in our gut, our microbiome. Researchers refer to the "gut–skin axis" to describe the complex relationship between the two.[96] It's thought that when the gut microbiome is imbalanced, it can trigger an inflammatory response that affects the skin, resulting in anything and everything – from acne and eczema to increased sensitivity, collagen breakdown and accelerated ageing.[97]

Candida is a type of yeast that's found naturally in the gut. Yet when we eat a diet that's high in sugar, are exposed to high levels of stress or take antibiotics, candida levels can grow and turn into what's known as intestinal candidiasis. This causes inflammation, which sends your immune system into overdrive and may show up within your skin as sensitivity, redness and breakouts.[98] Likewise, excessive yeast has been linked with fungal acne.

Poor gut health can also lead to malabsorption of essential nutrients, meaning our cells simply don't get the fuel they need to function well. So, if you want your skin to stay healthy, you need your gut to stay healthy too.

Your Shopping List for Glowing Skin

Like most people, I don't have hours to spend preparing food for myself and my family. While fads (and so-called "super" ingredients) will come and go, eating well to fuel your skin and body should never be about obscure or expensive ingredients – or spending hours slaving away. Making a basic shopping list with a variety of different foods can help you create a simple foundation that saves you time and money. You don't have to buy them all at once; you can just pick and choose items in each category from your list week to week, then have some quick and easy meals and snacks that you can rely on – particularly when you're short on time.

Here's a quick list that includes some of my favourite sources of protein, carbohydrate, good fats, vitamins and minerals, to keep my skin healthy and glowing.

The vast majority of people are fine to eat these foods; however, some people have food sensitivities, so please do bear this in mind. Often, a cooked version can have a very different effect on the body to eating the same food raw. For example, I love raw tomatoes, but my stomach does not! I'm fine if they're cooked (and the same goes for apples).

Foods to put on your list

Essential amino acids

Eggs, cottage cheese, turkey, buckwheat, hemp and chia seeds, peas.

Peptides

Eggs, meat, shellfish, beans, lentils, soy beans, bone broth.

Essential fatty acids

Tuna (fresh tuna is better as canned often has the fats removed) mackerel, salmon, flaxseeds and walnuts, pecans, sunflower seeds.

Lipids (good fats)

Chia seeds, avocado, oily fish, nuts, seeds, olive oil.

Minerals

Find copper in shitake mushrooms, leafy greens and dark chocolate. Top up your zinc levels with pumpkin (and its seeds), sweet potato, shellfish, legumes (such as chickpeas and lentils) dairy, eggs and whole grains. Manganese can be found in oatmeal, brown rice, pineapple and bananas.

Other minerals to consider as part of a healthy diet include selenium (which is especially high in Brazil nuts), magnesium (leafy vegetables, dark chocolate, avocado), calcium (cheese, yoghurt, milk, leafy vegetables, nuts, seeds, salmon) iron (chickpeas, dried apricots, pumpkin seeds, spinach, beetroot) and silica (oats, bananas, green beans, cucumber).

Vitamin A

There are two forms of vitamin A – retinol and beta-carotene. Find retinol in meat and eggs. Beta-carotene can be found in orange fruit and vegetables like carrots, sweet potato, pumpkin, squash, apricots, tangerines and cantaloupe melon. Asparagus, kale and spinach are also good sources.

Vitamin B

Eggs, poultry, fish, brown rice, lentils, mushrooms, beans, sunflower seeds, almonds, leafy greens, avocado, citrus fruits.

Vitamin C

Watercress, kale, broccoli, Brussels sprouts, red pepper, tomatoes, citrus fruits, strawberries and kiwi.

Vitamin E

Seeds, nuts, olives, olive oil, wheat germ oil, rainbow trout, avocado.

Vitamin D

Oily fish like sardines, salmon and mackerel, red meat (in moderation), egg yolks and some fortified milks, spreads and breakfast cereals (avoid those with a high sugar content).

Resveratrol

Another powerful free radical scavenger. Find it in red grapes, red wine (again, in moderation!), raisins and acai berries.

Vitamin K

If you're suffering from dark under-eye circles, try increasing your intake of vitamin K-rich spring onions, asparagus, broccoli, spinach, lettuce, kiwi and cooked rhubarb.

Flavonoids

Onions, kale, red wine, green tea, brightly coloured fruits and vegetables such as plums, apples, cherries, blueberries and tomatoes.

Greens, greens and more greens

We're often told to eat a rainbow of different coloured fruit and vegetables. This is a great rule to live by. Leafy green vegetables, in particular, bring incredible skin benefits, so try and squeeze some into your diet every day. These include collard greens, kale and spinach – all rich in an antioxidant called zeaxanthin, which is thought to improve the skin tone. Broccoli and Brussel sprouts also contain high levels of vitamin K, which boosts blood circulation. Spinach is also a great source of much-needed iron and zinc, which helps reduce inflammation.

Pre-and Probiotics

Up your intake of good bacteria-friendly prebiotic foods (chicory, Jerusalem artichokes, garlic, onions, leeks) and those rich in probiotics (yoghurt, kefir, miso, kombucha, sauerkraut and green olives).

Fibre

We need both soluble fibre (oats, rice bran, nuts, seeds, apples, strawberries) and insoluble fibre (grains, seeds, whole wheat, wheat bran, cauliflower and beans) to feed the good bacteria in our gut and help maintain a healthy microbiome. Fibre also helps keep our bowel movements regular, maintains blood sugar levels and lowers cholesterol levels as we get older.

Anti-inflammatory seasonings

Herbs and spices not only make our home-cooked meals tastier, but many also bring anti-inflammatory benefits. Try adding rosemary, basil, mint, turmeric, ginger, black pepper, cayenne pepper and cardamom to your food on a regular basis.

Water

Aim to drink eight glasses of water (more if it's hot, you're exercising, or going through menopause) throughout the day. Gasping through a hot, sweaty commute then downing your daily quota in one go is all very well, but your body will pee most of it out rather than using it to good effect!

Foods to leave off your list

Keep things like white bread, fried food, processed meat, fizzy drinks and sugar-laden ice creams, cakes, sweets and desserts off your regular shopping list. Sugar, in particular, has been linked to increased inflammation, acne and premature ageing. So, try only buying these foods from time to time.

Alcohol and caffeine are both broken down in the liver, and some people can tolerate more than others; we all have a genetic predisposition as to how our bodies cope with these. I know from having a DNA test that my body doesn't cope well with caffeine. If your skin is sensitive, dry, dull or flushing easily, with redness becoming standard, consider cutting one or both for at least three months to see if things improve.

Those prone to acne and dry skin conditions like eczema may want to try replacing dairy foods with other good sources of calcium. Likewise, gluten is often a trigger for digestive disorders. In which case, you might want to avoid foods such as bread, pasta, couscous, pizza and cooking sauces. All of these foods are now readily available in gluten-free versions. Please be aware that some of the gluten alternatives are packed with sugars that might aggravate your skin and body in other ways. I avoid most store-bought gluten-free breads as they make me feel bloated.

A NOTE ON HISTAMINES

While there is a growing focus on fermented ingredients which can be beneficial for our gut health, these types of foods can spark a histamine response (in the same way that your body might respond to an intolerance or allergy), resulting in redness, inflammation and rosacea. Not only have I experienced this, but some of my clients have too. Taking anti-histamine medication can confirm whether these foods are triggering a histamine response. Other foods that are high in histamines include dark chocolate, wine, dried fruit, avocado, spinach, shellfish and smoked meats.

My 70/30 rule for glowing skin

A lifetime of deprivation is hardly going to spark joy, and in fact, denying yourself your favourite treat will probably mean you're more likely to splurge the second you get your hands on it! Aim to include foods from the shopping list above in your diet for 70 per cent of the time, then give yourself permission to indulge in other foods for the remaining 30 per cent.

The Best Beauty Supplements

In the early days of my career, skin supplements weren't widely talked about. Fast forward fifteen years, and I'm inundated with new supplement launches every month! It's great to be able to top up our diet, but with so many options available, it can be hard to know which supplements are right for you and your skin.

Antioxidants

Almost every skin supplement will feature antioxidants as a means of helping your body repair the damage of oxidative stress.

Antioxidants to look out for:

Vitamin B3 (niacinamide): this ingredient has been around for decades, but has recently stolen the spotlight among beauty journalists and skin experts. A 2015 study showed that it may be helpful in the prevention of skin cancer. Others demonstrated its ability to limit oil production and reduce inflammation, making it a great all-round supplement for age prevention, acne, dry skin, rosacea and those with eczema.[99]

Vitamin C (often listed as ascorbic acid): helps our skin retain more moisture and supports collagen synthesis to keep our complexion looking smooth, plump and youthful.

Vitamin D (look for D3): in my view, almost everyone should be taking a supplement of the sunshine vitamin. Unlike other nutrients, which are often quantified in mg, Vitamin D3 is measured in IU (international units). It works particularly well with calcium and magnesium.

Vitamin E (look for d-alpha tocopherol, dl-alpha tocopherol and gamma tocopherol): this powerful antioxidant and anti-inflammatory supports the immune system, cell function and overall skin health, helping to protect against UV damage. Vitamins C and E complement each other but just be mindful not to overdo Vitamin E as it can be toxic.

Coenzyme Q10 (listed as CoQ10): this anti-ageing powerhouse has been shown to reduce the appearance of fine lines and wrinkles, increasing the thickness of the dermis and smoothing the skin texture overall.[100]

Lycopene: as an antioxidant found in tomatoes, lycopene can help increase your skin's defence against environmental ageing from UV radiation and pollution. Used in tandem with topical sunscreen, it's a great way of protecting your skin from premature ageing – inside and out.

Hydrators

Hyaluronic acid: as we age, the amount of this "miracle" hydrator within our skin falls. Synthesized hyaluronic acid supplements can counter this effect, reducing wrinkle depth and improving skin suppleness in just three months.[101]

Fats

Ceramides: as we know, these lipids play a vital role in maintaining our skin's structure and barrier function. One study showed that ceramide supplements obtained from wheat extract significantly increased hydration levels in women who suffered from very dry skin.[102]

Omegas 3 and 6: help maintain the skin barrier, reduce inflammation (helping to soothe dry skin, eczema and acne) and promote the all-important wound-healing processes.[103]

Collagen

Collagen peptides: if you'd asked me whether collagen supplements were worth it five years ago, I'd have told you not to waste your time and money! However, there's now scientific evidence to suggest that they can be effective. As a large molecule, collagen can't be absorbed by the small intestine. However, "hydrolyzed" collagen or "collagen peptides", which have been broken down into smaller molecules, can be absorbed more easily.[104] In doing so, they may help reduce the appearance of wrinkles, improve skin elasticity and boost moisture levels, giving us a plump, glowing complexion.

Marine collagen: collagen peptides derived from fish also have a low molecular weight and have been shown to improve skin elasticity and hydration levels. Fish collagen may support bone, joint and muscle health, which is particularly important as we age.[105]

Minerals

Selenium: this potent antioxidant helps prevent free radical damage and UV ageing, reducing inflammation, redness and sensitivity as long as it's taken in moderation – too much can be an issue. These types of minerals I much prefer taking when combined in formulations with other ingredients rather than as singular nutrients.

Magnesium (check the label for magnesium citrate, which is one of the most readily absorbed forms): as many as 70 per cent of the UK population could be deficient in this vital mineral, which is involved in more than 300 enzymatic reactions within the body.[106] Deficiency may show up on your skin as dryness, an uneven tone and fine lines.

MSM (methylsulfonylmethane): with its powerful anti-inflammatory properties, this sulphur-containing compound has traditionally been used to treat joint pain, muscle soreness and even arthritis. However, more recently, it has been used to support keratin (the main structural protein within our skin) and help us achieve a firmer, smoother complexion.[107]

Zinc (different forms include zinc gluconate, zinc sulphate and zinc picolinate): zinc is needed to make collagen and can help control inflammation. Zinc sulphate has been shown to help relieve acne; zinc gluconate is probably one of the most common forms, but zinc picolinate may be better absorbed.

Silica (look for bamboo extract and horsetail on labels): while this important mineral can get overlooked, it remains essential for healthy skin. Silica forms the building blocks of collagen[108] and helps the skin retain water, helping to relieve dryness and conditions like eczema and psoriasis.[109]

Prebiotics, probiotics and symbiotics

Probiotics are beneficial bacteria, and prebiotics are organisms that feed those good bacteria. Symbiotics contain both. When looking for probiotics, supplements should have around 1 billion colony-forming units (CFUs) and contain Lactobacillus, Bifidobacterium or Saccharomyces boulardii – some of the most well-researched bacterial strains. Prebiotics are often listed as galacto-oligosaccharides, fructo-oligosaccharides, oligofructose, chicory fibre and inulin.

How to pick a good supplement

Sadly, this is not an exact science. A long and complex list of factors come into play when we think about supplements. We're all different, so how effective a supplement will be can depend on how your body interacts with it, how bioavailable (readily absorbed) the nutrients are, and the quality of ingredients.

As a rule of thumb, avoid supplements containing the following fillers, which are often added to poor-quality supplements but hold no skin benefits: magnesium stearate, silicon dioxide, titanium dioxide, starch, microcrystalline cellulose, stearic acid, simethicone, vegetable gum, talc and propylene glycol. Likewise, you may want to select supplements that are vegan and/or free from sugar, gluten, soy and dairy, according to any intolerances.

Remember that supplements aren't silver bullets – they need time and consistency to work. So be patient, and you will get your skin glowing again!

A NOTE ON
IRON DEFICIENCY

Within the fast-moving supplement industry, iron is hardly a trending ingredient. But as it is the most abundant trace mineral within the body, particularly for women – whose iron levels are affected by our monthly cycles – it deserves a special mention.

Until we reach menopause, females bleed on a monthly basis, some more heavily than others. Whether you see your periods as a gift of life or a bit of a pain, it's worth taking a moment to think about how they change as we age – and how this affects our skin health.

Over time, our periods can become heavier. So, even if you've spent a lifetime without the merest sign of iron deficiency (anaemia), you may find your iron levels dip below normal as you get older.

The knock-on effect is huge – not least for the skin. Iron deficiency lowers the level of haemoglobin in the blood, which may reduce the amount of oxygen available to our cells. When the skin is deprived of oxygen, it can become dry and less resilient to intrinsic and extrinsic ageing.

Within my clinic, it's a combination of things I have learnt over the years that indicate a low iron level. The person's skin looks dull, sluggish, pale and tired, and doesn't respond to touch in a normal manner. Whenever this happens, I always delve a little deeper to find out how someone is feeling, both physically and emotionally. If I suspect there might be an iron deficiency, I'll suggest a visit to their GP for a blood test.

Be aware that calcium supplements, along with milk, caffeine and antacid tablets, can reduce the absorption of iron. So, be sure to leave at least two hours between those foods/medications and your iron supplement. Taking a vitamin C supplement at the same time has been shown to enhance iron absorption. And as a general rule, unless you know you need it, take iron in balance.

Get Your Glow – At Every Age

Lines and wrinkles are a part of who we are. We can't erase them completely – and neither should we want to. What we can focus on is maintaining healthy skin that has a healthy glow. When our skin looks fresh, plump and radiant, we feel great – no matter how old we are. A few dietary tweaks can make all the difference when it comes to making this happen.

My tips for balancing hormonal skin and restoring your glow:

- Increase your intake of essential fats: these help mitigate the effects of declining oestrogen levels to keep your skin plump. Try smoked salmon, avocado, walnuts, sunflower, flax, sesame and pumpkin seeds.

- Eat hormone-balancing foods: beans, oats, fennel, celery, parsley and rhubarb all contain phytoestrogens (plant oestrogens).

- Ensure you're getting enough calcium to support your bones and facial structure. Dairy products, fish with bones (sardines and mackerel) and dark leafy vegetables are an excellent place to start.

- Include protein with every meal: it'll provide your body with the amino acids it needs to support your skin, bones and muscles.

- If you're getting hot flushes, cut down on caffeine, alcohol and spicy food, as these can exacerbate your symptoms.

- Sleep, exercise and reduced stress levels are also your best friends when you're feeling the effects of hormonal changes. Yoga can be particularly helpful if you're struggling with anxiety, mood, fatigue or insomnia.

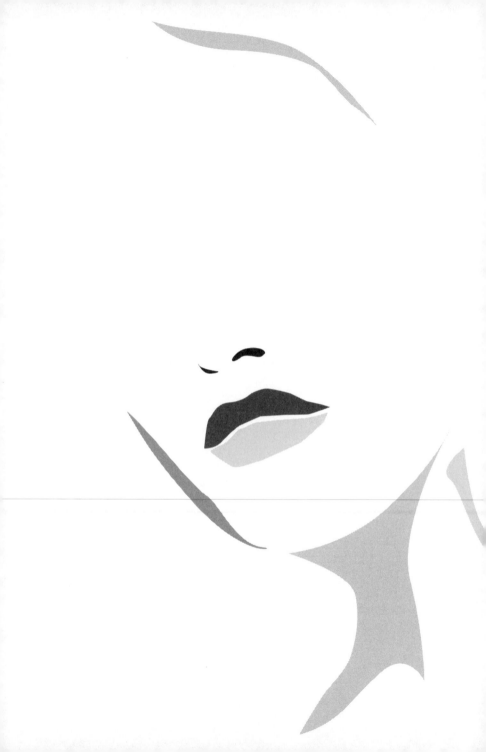

6

Skincare Basics

Building your Routine to Age Well

I didn't get my love for skincare from my mother – she was an E45 cream type of lady. Growing up in the 80s and 90s we didn't have the Internet to be kept up to date with the latest skincare trends and launches. We learnt from magazines or by visiting chemists or beauty salons.

It wasn't until my early twenties that I really began to understand skincare better and that was due to studying beauty therapy at night school, and frankly even that now seems quite limited in comparison to the knowledge I have gained over the years and also the information that is out there now. My first salon job taught me that expensive skincare ranges might not be the holy grail and that even they can cause skin reactions and breakouts and give very little result. It was this stark early experience that shaped the rest of my career, further study and research into more natural alternatives and effective, science-based skincare that supports the skin while giving results.

Our home skincare routine is essential. Every year, science and technology evolve to enable brands to create different, and in some cases more effective, formulations. Yet, the sheer number of new products launching means that the information we receive is not only overwhelming but often contradictory. Much of this information is bound up with marketing jargon and potentially over-hyped promises. And too often, we fall into the trap of thinking that more expensive means better or that it's gone viral on social media so it must be good. This is certainly not the case. In reality, a long list of factors – including your skin type, your age, the quality and concentration of the ingredients and how your products are formulated – will determine the results you get.

I know from treating thousands of faces that building the right home skincare routine is essential if you want your skin to be happy and to age well. A well-curated home-care regimen should work in tandem with any professional treatments you have (we'll come to those later). If in-clinic treatments prove too expensive or you just don't have the time or access to the right professionals, then the products you use morning and night – day in, day out – will form the bedrock of your facial care. I have witnessed this first-hand via my virtual consultations with people around the world – by following my skincare and wellbeing advice they have dramatically improved their skin condition, without even visiting me for a treatment.

In this chapter, we'll look at skincare routines, home gadgets and the latest technology with fresh eyes. So, if you woke up this morning and noticed your skin looking tired, dull or older than your years, let's get you back on track and recover your glow.

The Language of Skincare

Like many industries, the beauty sector comes with its own terminology. Understandably, it can all feel like a bit of a minefield. Use this quick checklist to familiarize yourself with some keywords and phrases that often crop up on product labels.

Clinically proven

It would be nice to think that, (as the term suggests), this refers to a product that's been through rigorous scientific trials on a large number of testers. Sadly, this is not the case. This term gives no indication of the methodology used or of the scale of a study. Clinical test results are hard to get hold of, so if a product does make this claim, see if it tells you how many people participated in the trial.

Dermatologically tested

This implies that a formulation has been tested for safety and efficacy on human skin under the watchful eye of dermatologists. Again, this is a nice idea, but without current legal regulation to support it, it means almost nothing.

Non-comedogenic

A "comedone" is the technical name for a type of pimple that results from a clogged pore. So "non-comedogenic" refers to products that won't block pores, making it a good choice for those prone to breakouts and acne. If you do suffer from these conditions, looking for non-comedogenic products is a good place to start. However, the term is unregulated, and there is no guarantee that products labelled in this way won't block pores.

Hypoallergenic

If you see this term on the label, it means it's relatively unlikely to cause an allergic reaction (the "hypo" refers to it presenting a lower than average risk). What it's not is allergy proof. Some hypoallergenic products even contain irritants like fragrance. As with other terminology, there's no legally binding standard, so you're better off checking a label for our list of potentially irritating ingredients and being especially mindful if you have medical allergies.

Active ingredient

Broadly, these are the ingredients that perform the function advertised on the front of the label ("brightening", "lifting" or "smoothing", for example). We'll come to specific actives in a moment, but as a general rule, ingredients are listed in order of concentration. This means that you want your actives to be at the top of the ingredients list, not way down near the bottom. "Inactive ingredients" typically refer to the delivery method used within the formula to transport the actives to where they need to be within the skin.

The Building Blocks of Your Home Routine

There's an overwhelming choice of cleansers, serums, toners, mists, exfoliators and creams out there – and more products launch all the time. The average woman is reported to spend around £570 a year on skincare,[110] yet more than 80 per cent of us are confused by this product category![111] I know I personally spend A LOT more than that.

It's easy to get swept up by the next big trend (a new "hero" ingredient or celebrity-endorsed anti-wrinkle cream). Rather than get seduced by the spin, let's start looking at some key ingredients and product types that form the building blocks of a good skincare routine. But please don't get too hung up on individual ingredients; I see this a lot and it can be counterproductive. Single ingredients are fine, but the key is a well-formulated combined product.

Cleansers

Cleansers come in the forms of milks, foams, gels, oils and balms. They're perhaps the most unglamorous product category and, as a result, can be underestimated. But cleansing is the most important part of your skincare routine! Get it wrong, and you can actually *create* a skin condition you didn't have before.

Yet, unless you find a product that effectively removes make-up, oil, sweat and bacteria – along with all that pollution from the day (without stripping) – then any product you apply afterwards won't be able to work as effectively as it should. Cleansing is also the first step in your facial massage routine. So, a good cleanser is vital if you want your skin to age well.

Most cleansers contain a surfactant (detergent): a chemical or natural compound that breaks through the surface tension of the skin to draw out dirt, oil, dead cells and pollution. These particles are removed as you rinse.

Traditional foaming cleansers can contain sodium lauryl sulphate (one of our irritants), so may make your skin more sensitive; brands are now swaying away from this, which is good news. Creams and milks generally offer a more soothing cleanse; balms often contain nourishing oils that "melt away" impurities and can be removed with a damp muslin cloth. Ideally, avoid balms containing mineral oil and paraffin. It's also now commonplace to see cleansers with added acids to exfoliate the skin while you're cleansing; some of these can be great if you have thicker, oilier skin but on a daily basis, morning and night might be too much.

As a guide, if your cleanser leaves your skin feeling tight and squeaky clean, it's a sign that it's too harsh for your skin, or frankly, not a very good formulation.

If you can afford to have two different types of cleanser then that's always my preference. Our skin is doing different things over a month with our changing hormones and environment: sometimes our skin might benefit from an exfoliating wash and at other times need something more soothing and hydrating to cleanse with.

Serums

Serums are your active ingredient powerhouse. They're designed to deliver a high concentration of ingredients directly into your skin, so it's worth spending some money on them. You can use different serums (and even layer serums) according to your skin type or problem. Serums can come in many different forms and because of this can be a little confusing. Oil, gel, water or lotion give them a liquid consistency that is best applied before thicker moisturizing creams and sunscreen. They're quickly and efficiently absorbed.

Day serums: these are usually all about protecting and hydrating the skin and/or targeting a specific skin concern. Many contain antioxidants such as vitamin C to brighten, hyaluronic acid to hydrate and vitamin E to protect against the effects of pollution.

Night serums: the primary function of a night serum is to either resurface, restore and repair skin. Like day serums, they should bring a high concentration of active ingredients in a lightweight formula that's readily absorbed and is applied after cleansing but before moisturizer or night oil or balm. Retinoids or Bakuchiol serums are also applied at night to support repair and regeneration.

Night-time is ideal to fit some sort of exfoliating glycolic, lactic, salicylic acid or more gentle mandelic acid into your routine; this might be done via a serum or an exfoliating tonic. Ingredients such as hyaluronic acid, niacinamide, azelaic acid (for acne and brightening), kojic acid (for lightening pigmentation) can be applied in the morning and/or at bedtime.

Tonics

These are not to be confused with toners (which have traditionally been used to restore the skin's pH after cleansing). Tonics are optional but can be a nice addition to your routine if you have particularly dry skin. Tonics (also referred to as "essences") often contain hydrating, nourishing and antioxidant ingredients like hyaluronic acid, aloe vera, rosewater, herbs and cucumber. Unlike toners, they remain on the skin rather than being wiped off. Please be aware that there are many variants when it comes to tonics and toners – some are great, others are not.

Ingredient highlight: hyaluronic acid

Arguably, hyaluronic acid is one of the most well-known skin hydrators. A polysaccharide (a sugar rather than an actual acid), it's found naturally within our bodies, predominantly in the skin, eyes and joints. It's seen as something of a miracle ingredient for its ability to hold up to 1,000 times its weight in moisture within skin cells. In my experience, it's well tolerated by most skin types (not all) and delivers fast (albeit temporary) results by plumping the skin. I have experienced some clients who find it irritates while it's absorbing; this is often when the skin is dehydrated and needs other hydrators such as ceramides. To make the most of your hyaluronic-acid serum, apply it to damp skin, then use your moisturizer straight afterwards to seal in hydration.

Retinoids

These are products containing ingredients derived from vitamin A. As one of the most firmly established anti-ageing ingredients, vitamin A promotes collagen production, supports cell regeneration, fades age spots, unclogs blocked pores, smooths a rough skin texture and generally helps your skin look and behave as if it's younger. They have become some of the most talked about skincare ingredients and are put on something of a pedestal. I love them, but in my professional opinion they are not essential to gain fantastic results.

Retinyl palmitate: a great place to begin because it's gentler and less irritating than other retinoids. Bear in mind that it's not a dermal collagen stimulator, so while it does work to plump the skin, it acts on a more superficial level, rather than delivering results deep down.

Retinal: this is a slightly different form of vitamin A. It's more gentle than retinol and has a greater impact on long-term collagen production. It's one I feel brands should focus on more than just retinol.

Retinol: over the counter, it comes in serum and cream form and is available in various strengths (the most common being 0.25 per cent, 0.5 per cent, 1 per cent and 2 per cent). Anything less than 0.25 per cent is unlikely to deliver real results.

On prescription: retinol is available in much stronger concentrations in the form of Tretinoin (for the treatment of acne and pigmentation) and Roaccutane (a form of vitamin A that's taken orally for severe acne).

Retinoids should be applied at night to allow for maximum absorption. Avoid them while pregnant and in places where UV levels are high.

It's worth noting that retinoids can cause redness, peeling and sensitivity when you start, as it takes a while for the skin to get used to them. Retinol can remain in the skin for up to thirty-six hours, so even if you apply it at night, be sure to use SPF in the morning to protect against sun damage. It's best to start with a lower concentration and apply your retinol a couple of times a week before increasing the dose and frequency gradually over the course of several weeks or months.

Bakuchiol

Again, not a product type, but a newer ingredient that's often used as a natural alternative to retinol because it follows some of the same skin-improving pathways. A vegan ingredient derived from Chinese medicine, it's effective on all skin types. Bakuchiol can help restore firmness, reduce lines and refine the skin tone and texture. With its soothing properties, it's great for people who are prone to sensitivity and acne, is safe for use during pregnancy and can be used alongside retinol.

Moisturizers

Occlusives: these mimic the skin's natural lipids and form a protective barrier to prevent moisture loss – a bit like a waterproof coat. They're useful in treating very dry skin. Common natural occlusives include shea butter, argan and jojoba oil. Although Vaseline is another well-known occlusive, it seals the skin, rather than adding moisture. Prolonged use of Vaseline can cause dehydration, dullness and breakouts, so I'd only ever recommend using it for a short period when treating severely dry skin conditions.

Humectants: humectants attract and transport moisture into the skin. Hyaluronic acid is a humectant, as is glycerine and urea. Like occlusives, you'll find them in leave-on products such as serums, lotions and face creams.

Emollients: emollients have some occlusive and humectant properties. They work to soften the skin and restore that vital barrier function and are often listed as esters (waxes and oils), fatty acids and lipids (linoleic and oleic acid, as well as squalene and squalane) and cholesterols. The latter make up around 25 per cent of the skin's lipid barrier, making them an essential – but often overlooked – skincare component. You can find them in gels, creams, balms and ointments.

Ceramides: like cholesterols, ceramides are vital for maintaining your skin barrier. The lipid "mortar" within the skin barrier is made up of ceramides (fats) which keep the structure together but (no surprise) decline as we age. They form a protective, plumping layer that locks in moisture and keeps your skin looking youthful. The ceramides found in skincare products closely resemble those found naturally within the skin, making them highly effective. Soothing moisturizers often contain ceramides. Likewise, they're often found in gentle cleansers, which are a great way of removing impurities while supporting your skin barrier.

Chemical exfoliants and home peels

The function of an exfoliator is to remove dead cells, dirt and impurities from the skin's surface. Exfoliation smooths the skin texture and makes way for healthy new cells. You can find them in the form of serums, toners and home peels – which are left on for a period of time, like a mask, before rinsing. Using them once or twice a week is generally sufficient for most people. Different acids bring different benefits:

Alpha-hydroxy Acids (AHAs): these include lactic acid (helps increase skin moisture levels); glycolic acid (very effective but can cause sensitivity); mandelic acid (great for oily skins as it has antibacterial properties); azelaic acid (ideal for breakouts and smoothing the skin texture) and kojic acid (for fading pigmentation). These acids have a medium molecular weight (or size) that allows them to act on the middle layers of the skin.

Beta-hydroxy Acids (BHAs): these are most commonly found in skincare in the form of salicylic acid. This acid has a low molecular weight, allowing it to penetrate deep into the skin and clean out clogged pores. It has both anti-inflammatory and antibacterial properties, making it useful for those with breakouts and acne.

Polyhydroxy Acids (PHAs): these include lactobionic acid and gluconolactone. They work in a similar way to AHAs but have a higher molecular weight, so work on a more superficial level, making them less irritating. They help strengthen the skin barrier and reduce the signs of ageing with minimal side effects, so they're ideal for dry and sensitive skin types.

Masks

Masks are an integral part of any professional facial for a reason: a good mask that's targeted to your particular skin concerns can have transformative results. Yes, they take up a little more of your time. But in addition to their evident skin benefits, building masks into your home routine is a lovely way to relax and take some time out from your busy day. Like serums, masks are usually packed with a high concentration of ingredients. I love to apply them before a social event, when I want my skin to have an extra glow.

For plumping: as we age and collagen and oestrogen levels decline, look for plumping, hydrating masks containing hyaluronic acid, ceramides, peptides, fatty acids (argan, marula or safflower oil), soothing aloe vera and moisturizing shea butter.

To brighten and restore your glow: if you want to reduce the appearance of age spots and tighten skin, look for masks containing AHAs, BHAs, kojic acid, liquorice, vitamin C, ginseng, fruit enzymes and sea algae.

Minerals and mists

Minerals don't just keep our body healthy, they also help our skin function well. Potassium and sodium work to retain cell water levels, magnesium and silicone maintain cells' integrity, magnesium can help reduce oxidative stress and breakouts, calcium supports tissue healing, while copper is needed for collagen and elastin production. They're often included in skincare in the form of mineral-rich "thermal water" or facial sprays.

A NOTE ON COLLAGEN CREAMS

We all know how important collagen is if we're to maintain healthy, youthful-looking skin. We also know that collagen production stalls as we age. Yet, while it might seem tempting to counteract this decline with a collagen cream, we need to be realistic about their results. Collagen molecules within skincare are simply too large to penetrate the skin or deliver any direct collagen stimulation. That said, collagen cream can work well as means of making the skin appear plumper and better hydrated on the surface.

Oils and Balms

Oils and oil-based balms bring amazing skin-nourishing benefits, and they're also the foundation of your facial massage plan. The nature of their texture allows them to provide "slip" that stops you from dragging and damaging your skin. By massaging them in, you're also helping them penetrate the skin more effectively.

However, not all oils are created equal – and some cause breakouts. As a general rule, avoid products containing petrolatum, mineral oil, beeswax, lanolin and paraffin, as they might clog pores and trigger spots.

As fats, oils are a brilliant way of helping to restore and fortify the lipid-rich skin barrier. Plant oils have also been shown to bring anti-inflammatory and antibacterial benefits while promoting wound healing and increasing collagen synthesis.[112] Some plant oils to look out for when building your skin routine are:

For dry/sensitive skin: sweet almond, peach kernel, evening primrose, St John's wort and avocado oil.

For anti-ageing benefits: argan, rosehip seed, camellia, sea buckthorn, pomegranate seed oil.

For oily skin: don't assume that you should avoid facial oils altogether. If the skin finds it has too little oil, it can send sebum production into overdrive, worsening breakouts and acne. Instead, look for "dry oils" which have a lighter texture, mimic the skin's natural oils and absorb more easily. Such oils include moringa, safflower, hemp, borage, rosemary and milk thistle.

For pre-make-up: applying a facial oil before make-up has got a bad reputation. Many women fear it will make them look shiny, reduce the wear of their make-up or cause their foundation to pill. Actually, a morning massage is a fantastic way to encourage lymphatic drainage and reduce puffiness. The following oils are quickly absorbed and will give you a glow – without disturbing your make-up: marula, moringa, grapeseed oil and squalene.

As oils tend to have larger molecules than serums or retinol, it's a good idea to apply them afterwards. This will allow your antioxidants to penetrate deep into the skin before you apply your chosen oil.

———————————

Sunscreen – Your Anti-ageing Super Product

For some reason, many people still see sunscreen as something they need to apply on a sunny day or while on holiday. This couldn't be further from the reality. In acting as a filter against UV radiation and pollution, sunscreen is a vital element of our daily skincare routine. And yes, that does mean in winter too (forget waiting for sunny days; if it's light outside, you need sunscreen).

In order for SPF to be effective, you need to apply a decent amount (at least enough to cover the length of two fingers when you squeeze it out of the bottle). It also needs to cover your whole face – not just the bits you think might burn, like the bridge of your nose and cheekbones.

Sunscreens have come a long way from the days of thick, white creams that left a ghostly mask on your skin. New textures and technologies mean that many formulations now absorb quickly, sit invisibly beneath make-up and won't make your eyes sting. There are two main types of sunscreen:

Chemical sunscreens: might contain octocrylene, avobenzone, oxybenzone and helioplex. These work to *absorb* UV rays, triggering a chemical reaction that activates their protective capabilities to "break down" sunlight.

Mineral or "physical" sun protectors: these form a defensive shield. They commonly contain the minerals zinc oxide and titanium dioxide to *block* UVA and UVB rays. These minerals have mild healing properties, so are excellent for those with sensitive or acne-prone skin.

SPF (sun protection factor): refers to how long a particular product will offer protection against the sun, versus the time it would take to burn if you hadn't applied it. So, theoretically, it should take thirty times longer for your skin to redden if you're wearing an SPF 30 than if you haven't applied any at all. However, don't be fooled into thinking that using a high SPF means you can sunbathe safely for longer. The reality is that no product offers fool-proof protection, and whatever your age or skin type, sitting in direct sunlight for hours on end will damage your skin and accelerate ageing.

The PA+ symbol: refers to a rating system developed in Japan to represent how much UVA protection a product offers. PA+ means there is some moderate UVA protection; PA++ means a little more and PA++++ delivers extremely high protection against UVA rays. It has to be said, there are question marks over this rating (and how to standardize it across different countries), so it's not essential.

Day cream or sunscreen?

I often get asked if we need a separate sunscreen if our day cream has an SPF on the label. While it might be tempting to kill two birds with one stone, I always use a separate moisturizer and SPF. A recent study by Liverpool University found that an SPF 30 moisturizer did not match the level of protection offered by an SPF 30 sunscreen.[113] So, if your skin is dry, apply a good moisturizer. Then use a separate sunscreen to protect you from UV-related ageing.

———————————

Skincare on a Plate

How our skin looks and feels is also intrinsically linked with how we feel about ourselves. More than 50 per cent of women say that skin problems hold them back from living life to the full.[114]

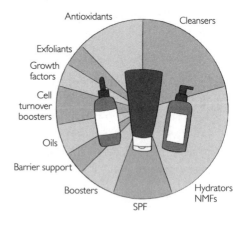

Remember that your skin is as unique as your genetics. So, what works for your friend – with different genetics, who lives in a different place and has a different lifestyle to you – may not be the best product for you. The best way to start thinking about a routine that's right for your skin is to imagine a plate of food. Just as we know that our diet should be made up of *at least* five portions of fruit and veg a day (ideally more!) along with protein, healthy fats and whole grains, we can imagine certain ingredients on a plate. Together – and in the right balance – they form a perfectly balanced skin plan for you.

Layering Your Skincare Products

Unlike the food we put on our plate, which we can eat in any way or order we fancy, there's a system to applying and layering your skin products. The rules below aren't set in stone, but they do provide a useful guide so that each product can work effectively and give you the best possible results. In general, work from thinner consistencies up toward thicker ones.

Morning:

1. Cleanser

2. Toner (optional)

3. Serum (thinnest first if you're using more than one)

4. Eye cream

5. Moisturizer

6. Sunscreen

Evening:

1. Cleanser

2. Exfoliant (optional)

3. Toner (optional)

4. Serum/retinoid

5. Moisturizer/oil/balm/second serum

I'm not a huge fan of heavy creams at night. I have seen time and time again that this doesn't suit all skin types, especially those prone to oiliness and breakouts; I much prefer to layer serums, tonics and oils in the evening.

Your Questions Answered

In all my years working with clients, some questions crop up time and time again. Here are some of the most commonly asked questions about building a great skincare routine at home.

1. Do I need to double cleanse – morning and night?

No. You should cleanse in the morning as well as at night. The skin secretes certain toxins overnight, so a morning cleanse will remove unwanted impurities and prepare your skin for your daytime products, so they can work more effectively.

As for double cleansing – it depends! Not all skin types need to double cleanse, and it depends on how much make-up you wear, etc. If you have dry, sensitive skin, one round with a hydrating cleanser removed gently with a soft muslin cloth and tepid (not hot!) water should be sufficient.

If you do want to double cleanse, you can use a cleanser to remove the uppermost make-up and surface grime, then perform a second round to give your skin a more thorough cleanse deep down. I like to use a cream or balm the first time and a gentle wash for the second.

2. Is micellar water the same as a toner?

No! Micellar waters can be used as a pre-cleanse step in your skincare routine. They take their name from "micelles", which are tiny round balls of cleansing oil molecules that float in water and attract impurities like a magnet when you swipe them over the skin with a cotton pad. Micellar waters can be a good, gentle way to cleanse sensitive and eczema-prone skin.

Toners, on the other hand, were traditionally a means of removing a cream cleanser. They were often loaded with alcohol that stripped the skin. Depending on your skin type, you could use a hydrating toner or something more balancing.

3. Should all my products be from the same range?

The idea that all your skincare should come from the same range is a clever marketing myth designed to keep you spending money on the same brand. It's perfectly okay to use products from different brands. It's much more important to think of your skincare routine as a whole, rather than focusing on specific ranges.

4. Can I use retinol with AHAs?

Yes! Retinol and exfoliators like alpha-hydroxy acids can work well together. While AHAs work nearer the surface, retinol works on a deeper layer of the skin, so in fact they complement each other. You may need to reduce your use of AHAs when you start using retinol to minimize irritation. Balance is key here, so listen to what your skin is telling you.

5. When should I start using "anti-ageing" products?

Ageing well isn't just about correcting and repairing damage – it's about preventing it. Collagen production and cell turnover slow down in our twenties, and we may begin to notice a few fine lines around our eyes. So, even at this age, we can build a balanced skincare regimen with products that keep our skin well-hydrated, protect the skin barrier and combat free radical damage to prevent ageing. Generally, high street "anti-ageing" products are thicker and richer which would be too much for a skin under the age of thirty-five. However I have many of my clients across all ages on similar cosmeceutical/pharma-grade skincare as their target is skin change not product thickness.

My Absolute No-no List

As everyone's skin is so different, I'm not usually one for hard and fast rules. That said, there are some things which I just never do – and advise my clients to steer clear of too.

Face wipes: loaded with alcohol and fragrance, wipes can strip the skin, compromise barrier function and cause inflammation and redness. Apart from the fact that they're convenient, they have no redeeming features for the skin. Most are made from a fabric mixed with plastic resins such as polyester or polypropylene, which don't break down and so end up in waterways. If you must use them for a short trip or festival, biodegradable wipes are now available.

Sheet masks: these have become a huge trend in recent years for their ability to deliver a concentrated dose of skin-beneficial ingredients in one hit. However, like face wipes, they're single-use, generally non-biodegradable and usually in non-recyclable packaging, so hardly planet-friendly. A traditional mask or good-quality serum is a better choice.

Anything highly synthetically fragranced: even if you can't see redness or sensitivity, they can cause damage deep down. Synthetic fragrance has no benefit at all to the skin – so avoid.

Sleeping in your make-up: no – this is not just an old wives' tale! By leaving dirt, make-up and daily pollution on your face at night, you're inhibiting the skin's natural repair mode and are likely to develop visibly clogged pores, breakouts, dryness and irritation. The oxidative stress caused by pollution particles could also accelerate free radical damage and skin ageing. Sleep in your make-up for just one night, and you'll notice the effects; do it regularly and you really will make your skin age faster.

Gadgets and Technology to Use at Home

Having worked on so many faces for so many years, I know how powerful and transformative professional treatments can be. While they used to consist of a series of products being applied to and removed from the skin, these days facials employ the latest technology and gadgetry to tackle all manner of skin issues and restore the skin's natural glow.

You can now also buy some good gadgets to use at home. For safety reasons and size of machinery they are less powerful than the machinery found in professional clinics; however using them regularly as part of your home-care routine can make a difference.

A key point to note: not all machines are the same. If it's cheap it's probably not likely to do much – you do pay for good technology. See it as an investment; you are going to get lots of use out of that one machine.

LED therapy

LED stands for light-emitting diode. The science and technology was originally NASA based, used to grow plant life in shuttle missions, so you could call it the face treatment from outer space. The machines emit light which gets absorbed by the skin and acts from there.

It's non-invasive, simple and safe to use and very effective if used regularly.

Each device might use different wavelengths of light. The most commonly used and universal is red light, which stimulates collagen and elastin production, increases blood flow and tissue oxygenation and leaves your skin looking plump and rejuvenated. A key point is also the number of lights used, which can impact on the price and effectiveness. Some machines have the addition of

Near Infrared (NIR) which is able to penetrate deeper and have a more profound response.

There is some evidence to suggest that low-intensity LED therapy also triggers the production of ATP. As we discovered in Chapter 3, when thinking about the benefits of physical activity, ATP is involved in repairing damage and making essential skin components like collagen and hyaluronic acid.

LED therapy is good for all skin types and conditions, including acne, redness, inflamed skin; reducing fine lines and wrinkles; dry, dull skin. It is safe to use 3–4 times a week.

Radiofrequency

At-home radiofrequency tools work in the same way as the machines used in professional treatments, but are much less powerful. Radiofrequency uses heat that travels beneath the skin surface to act within the dermis. Here, this energy stimulates elastin and collagen production to firm and tighten the skin, while protecting the uppermost layer. It's ideal if you want to tackle loose skin around the neck, jawline and chin.

Radiofrequency is good for firming and glow.

IPL

Intense Pulsed Light (IPL) is used to reduce the appearance of age spots, hyperpigmentation, rosacea, thread veins, acne, fine lines and wrinkles and as a means of hair removal. It works by targeting different colours within the skin. For skin rejuvenation it targets melanin (the pigment within your skin) or blood, vascular. Please note, because of the way it affects melanin, IPL is not suitable if you have a dark skin tone unless in the hands of a well-trained professional with specific clinic machinery. I love IPL in clinic; it is an incredible tool for skin rejuvenation. I have not to date found an effective at-home device.

Microcurrent

Microcurrent therapy is now available in small handheld devices the size of your phone and smaller. These gadgets work by sending different electrical currents into your skin to boost ATP, increasing cell energy, communication and repair and also supporting muscle tone. Over time, this stimulates the production of skin-plumping collagen and elastin.

You need to apply a conductive gel to the skin for the current to pass through. Some devices are much more effective than others. My current favourite at-home devices are the ZIIP device[115] and NuFACE.

Microcurrent is good for lifting, toning, hydration, general rejuvenation. It is safe to use 3–4 times a week.

Microneedling

Microneedling at home involves using a derma-roller or derma stamp covered with tiny fine needles. By rolling it over the skin, you create microscopic pinpricks, or what experts refer to as "controlled wounds". This action stimulates your skin's natural repair process, boosting collagen and elastin production. Microneedling also helps products be absorbed more effectively, so you get a kind of double-whammy effect – however, not all skincare is good to infuse; I only recommend specific serums and usually from a clean, cosmeceutical/pharma-grade source intended to work on and in the skin. Not high-street serums please – these are not suitable for advanced penetration.

It might sound painful, but the needles are tiny, around 0.25mm long for home derma-rollers, maximum length 0.5mm; clinic rollers are 0.5mm to 2mm. So while your skin may look a little flushed immediately afterwards, it doesn't hurt[116]. The key is not to overdo it or drag the roller – be gentle and sterilize between each use. Use once a week.

Microneedling is good for: glow, fine lines.

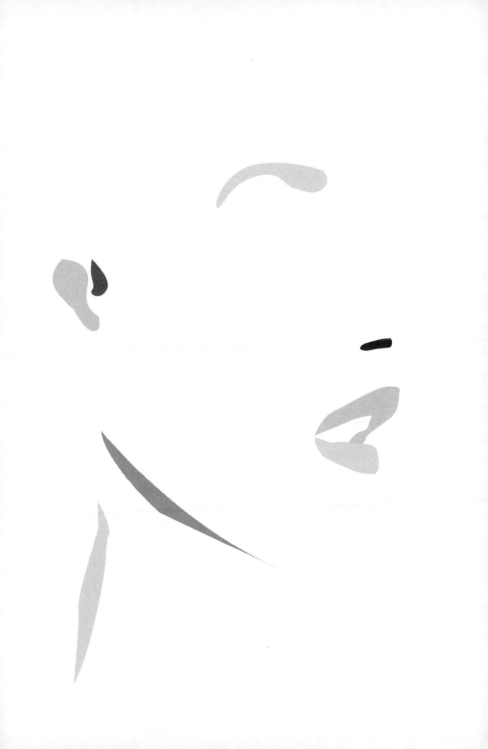

7

Skincare Anatomy

Training Your Face to Age Well

For as long as I can remember, I've been a firm believer in the power of touch. My formal education in massage took place at beauty college – I was lucky enough to receive the Holistic Therapist of the Year Award. Yet, while I was trained in everything from nails to waxing and tanning, it was the massage and facial modules – and the element of human touch – that I loved the most and that I took to intuitively.

As you'll know, a seemingly endless list of massage techniques exists – and you name it, I've studied it. Starting with Swedish and sports massage, I moved onto Vodder Manual Lymph Drainage (we'll come to this later), facial reflexology, myofascial release, Thai, Ayurvedic, Indian and Japanese face massage. I've even trained in pregnancy and baby massage. All these methods have similarities, yet are unique. Perhaps surprisingly, it was studying baby massage that had a profound effect on me. I learnt about the power of positive touch, the relationship between the giver and the receiver and how massage is used all around the world to alleviate mental as well as physical health conditions.

Later, I came across a book that undoubtedly changed the course of my career. *Touching: The Human Significance of the Skin* by British-American anthropologist Ashley Montagu was first published in 1971. Having begun to translate my knowledge of body massage techniques to the face, this book has shaped my practice with clients ever since. Over the years, I've witnessed first-hand how the muscles and tissues of the face can be transformed through the power of massage. And let's not forget the impact it has on our emotional wellbeing too. For all these reasons, facial massage, for me, really is a key component of glowing skin – and one of the secrets to ageing well.

Face massage is not just about rubbing creams into your face, however nice that might feel. It comes with specific techniques based on an in-depth knowledge of the tissues, muscles, lymph, fascia, collagen and elastin beneath the skin's surface. By learning how to manipulate these structures correctly, we can train our face to look younger – just as we exercise our body to keep it strong and healthy.

In this chapter, we'll dive deep into facial anatomy to understand how facial massage can unlock great skin at every age.

The 6 Functions of the Skin

To retrain our skin, we need to know what it does – and how it works. Our skin makes up 15 per cent of our total adult body weight and ranges in thickness from less than 0.1mm on our eyelids to 1.5mm on the palms of our hands and soles of our feet.[117] Across the body, the skin performs six essential functions.

1. **Protection:** from injury, harmful agents, UV radiation and moisture loss, acting as part of the immune system.

2. **Storage:** of lipids (fats) and water.

3. **Thermoregulation:** by producing sweat and dilating blood vessels, the skin keeps us cool. So-called "goosebumps" and

the constriction of blood vessels allow us to retain heat when we're cold.

4. **Sensation:** nerve endings detect temperature, pressure, vibration and injury, dictating how we experience touch, whether it's pleasurable or painful.

5. **Controlling water loss:** our skin prevents moisture from escaping via evaporation.

6. **Water resistance:** it also stops nutrients from being washed away.

Your Skin's Anatomy

The skin is made up of three main layers – the epidermis, the dermis and the hypodermis. Each of these contains complex sub-layers and structures.

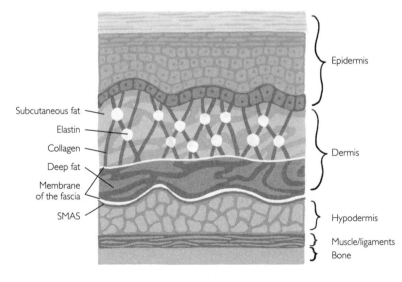

Epidermis: consists of the stratum corneum (the outmost layer), along with several sub-layers. The epidermis is mostly made up of cells called keratinocytes. It's where we find the all-important skin barrier, along with melanocytes, which produce pigment.

Dermo-epidermal junction: this is a double-layered structure that acts as an interface for oxygen, nutrients and waste products to be exchanged between the epidermis and dermis. As we discovered in Chapter 6, regular cosmetic products can't penetrate this junction. By contrast, the active ingredients within cosmeceuticals can do so, which explains why they're able to bring about physical changes within the skin.

Dermis: this thicker layer provides nourishment to the epidermis and plays an important part in wound healing. It consists of 70 per cent collagen, along with some elastin and specialized cells such as fibroblasts (which make collagen and elastin), blood vessels, lymphatics, sweat glands and nerves.

Hypodermis: located beneath the dermis, the hypodermis consists mainly of fat, along with blood vessels and nerves. It acts as a means of insulating the body from cold and aiding in shock absorption.

Collagen and Elastin

Think about a new mattress: when you first buy it, the springs are nice and firm. Over time, they lose their bounce and springiness; the mattress lacks support – and begins to sag. A similar thing happens within our skin as collagen and elastin production begins to slow from our twenties onward.

Collagen

Collagen is the substance that holds the body together. It's found in the bones, skin, muscles, connective tissues and is a major component in the outer eyeball. It's hard, insoluble, fibrous protein. In fact, collagen makes up a third of the protein within our bodies. It's thought that there are as many as sixteen different types of collagen, and in most cases, the molecules are packed together to form long, thin "fibrils".

Amazingly, "Type 1" collagen is, gram for gram, stronger than steel![118] In being so strong and flexible (just like the springs on your new mattress), collagen is what gives the skin its structure. Yet, as we age and are exposed to external stressors like pollution and UV radiation, collagen production falls. This decline is particularly steep following menopause. As a result, the skin structure is compromised, joint cartilage gets weaker and we develop wrinkles.

Elastin

Like collagen, elastin is a protein and it's found in tendons, arteries and lungs. It's another one of the main structural components within our skin. However, elastin is a different type of protein to collagen. It's about 1000 times more elastic (hence the name) and is the reason why young skin bounces back into place when you move it.[119]

As we age, elastin gets weaker, rather like an elastic band that has been stretched over and over again for many years. This repetitive stretching action shows up on our skin as we develop sagging – particularly around the eyes, jawline and neck.

Collagen and elastin work together to give our skin its shape and firmness. Collagen provides structure and rigidity; elastic gives it stretch, so we can move and show our emotions via our facial expressions, for example.

Fascia

Fascia is a hot topic for anyone interested in both body and facial fitness. Fascia is continuous three-dimensional matrix that wraps around the body like a figure-hugging suit. As a sheet of fibrous connective tissue made up of closely packed bundles of collagen, it's what links the muscles, bones, nerves and blood vessels together. It's amazingly strong and can hold a tensile pressure of 2,000 pounds per square inch.[120]

The natural ageing process, along with our increasingly sedentary, desk-bound lifestyles, means the fascia changes from a healthy "fluid" structure to one that's stiff or even "sticky". In the body, this can cause stiffness, pain and injury (hence why foam rollers and other myofascial release techniques have become popular). In the face, it can make us look older as our skin loses its structure, plumpness and glow.

On the face, there are two layers of fascia: the deep layer, which surrounds the muscles and is rich in elastin, blood vessels and sensory receptors; and the superficial layer, which sits in the bottom layer of skin.

Fascia is highly elastic and supports our skin, giving it lift and tone. As we age, our fascia moves from its original, youthful position and we develop lines and wrinkles. Yet, manipulating our fascia can unlock powerful anti-ageing skin benefits. Fascia is "thixotropic" – meaning that it can elongate and reset in a more favourable position when manipulated and released correctly. Using specific massage movements, we can lift the fascia back toward its former position, giving our face a more sculpted look.

Better still, because the superficial fascia serves as a storage place for fat and water – as well as a passageway for lymph – manipulating it can boost lymphatic drainage, helping to remove waste and deliver vital nutrients that keep our skin cells healthy.

Fat

Like fascia, facial fat is divided into two layers. Together, they help maintain the structure and plumpness of our skin. As we age, we tend to lose fat around the middle of our face (atrophy), causing us to lose volume and make our skin sag – especially around the eyes and cheeks. Conversely, we often gain fat (hypertrophy) in the lower part of our face, which leads to jowls. Many professional treatments work to offset this effect by rebalancing the facial proportions.

The SMAS

The SMAS – or superficial musculoaponeurotic system – is used to describe the middle and lower third of the face. One of its primary functions is to transmit, distribute and amplify the activity of our facial muscles.[121] The SMAS is what a surgeon works on when we have a facelift. By manoeuvring and tightening the SMAS layer, we can counter age-related drooping of fat to bring about overall facial rejuvenation.[122] So, your surgeon quite literally lifts the layer beneath the skin to mimic the structure of a younger face.

Lymphatics

Manual Lymphatic Drainage (MLD) sounds rather aggressive, but actually refers to an extremely "light touch" form of massage that encourages lymph flow.

Originating from the Latin word for water, lymph is a colourless fluid, predominantly made up of white blood cells, that attacks bacteria in the blood and removes waste products from our tissues. Lymph is transported by the body's lymphatic system: a network of delicate vessels that helps regulate fluid levels, filter bacteria, absorb fatty acids and produce white blood cells. It plays an important role in our immune system.

Lymph nodes – or glands – monitor lymph flow. The lymph nodes we stimulate during our facial massage are found near the base of the skull, and behind and in front of each ear. They also run down each side of our neck, appear beneath the jawline and chin and at the collarbone and in the armpits.

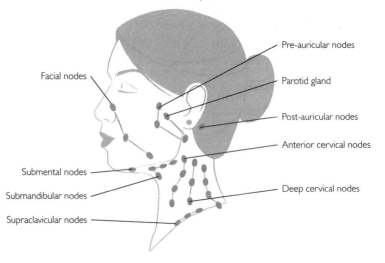

Facial nodes

Pre-auricular nodes

Parotid gland

Post-auricular nodes

Anterior cervical nodes

Submental nodes

Deep cervical nodes

Submandibular nodes

Supraclavicular nodes

Muscle

Unlike those of the body, our facial muscles don't all directly attach to bone. Rather, many of them attach under the skin so that they can fulfil two important roles: chewing and forming expressions. There are forty-two muscles in the face, which move when we smile, frown, blink, laugh, cry and emote in any number of ways. We blink anywhere between 14,400 and 19,200 times a day to protect and oxygenate our eyes,[123] so these muscles are both highly active and essential for our health.

Of course, muscle is also a place where we hold tension. Spending hours in a sitting position, looking down at our screen each day, compromises correct posture and can cause neck and shoulder pain (most of us have experienced the discomfort of "tech neck" at some point). Research shows that within just a few seconds of experiencing a negative emotion, we clench our jaw and tense the muscles around our eyes and mouth.[124]

Facial massage can release this muscular tension. Not only does this help our skin and face appear more rested and rejuvenated, but it can also make us feel more energized and happier too.

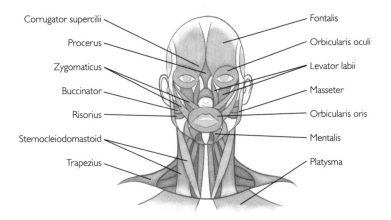

Corrugator supercilii
Procerus
Zygomaticus
Buccinator
Risorius
Sternocleiodomastoid
Trapezius

Fontalis
Orbicularis oculi
Levator labii
Masseter
Orbicularis oris
Mentalis
Platysma

Bones

The lines, wrinkles and sagging that develop over time are more than skin (and muscle) deep. As we age, our bones change shape. Our eye sockets get wider and longer, and the angles of the bones that form our brow, nose and jaw all decrease.[125] As women, the accompanying fall in oestrogen levels – particularly when we reach menopause – also leads to a loss of bone density.

As our bones are the "scaffolding" of our skin, the fall in density leads to skin sagging and loss of volume, which in turn leads to wrinkles. These changes in bone structure also mean that, even after having a facelift or injectables, we can never assume the appearance of our youth. These treatments only act on the skin, so it's essential to maintain good bone health throughout our lives via our diet, supplementation and safe sun exposure.

Your Skin Through the Decades

The face is amazing. A foetus begins to develop facial characteristics as early as four to six weeks into a pregnancy.[126] As one of the most variable structures in the body, its expressions shape our identity and inform how we're perceived by others. It fascinates me how as children we often take on similar facial expressions of our parents.

We know that changes in skin cell production, fat placement and bone structure are what make us appear older over time. In order to understand – and respond to – these changes, it's helpful to divide the face into three sections.

Upper face: runs from the hairline, down the forehead and across the temples, stopping just beneath the lower eyelids.

Middle face: starts at the lower eyelid and includes the cheeks, nose and ears.

Lower face: begins at the upper lip, ends at the lower border of the chin and includes the chin and lips.

Age affects the different facial areas in a variety of ways:

In your twenties: you have great collagen support, optimal cell turnover and plenty of fat cells, so your skin is plump and bouncy. Imbalances in sebum levels can cause acne and pimples, especially around the jawline. Many people have combination skin, which is oily and prone to blackheads around the T-zone (nose, cheeks and forehead) and dry on the cheeks. Start learning the principles of face massage now because, at this age, you don't need Botox or fillers!

In your thirties: as collagen levels decline and cell renewal slows, you may start noticing some fine lines, particularly around your eyes. If you have an expressive forehead or tend to frown a lot, lines may start to appear on the upper face and between the brows (glabellar lines). Our face can become slimmer and more angular as we begin to lose volume in the mid and lower face.

Uneven pigmentation, melasma (darker, discoloured patches) and chloasma (the butterfly-shaped "mask of pregnancy") will often accompany hormonal changes. Under-eye circles may darken, and you may also see a few broken capillaries pop up here and there.

In your forties: oestrogen levels decline, and our skin becomes less plump, hydrated and glowy. Collagen, elastin and hyaluronic acid levels within the skin are falling, and muscle tone begins to slacken. The fat pads in the upper and middle parts of the face experience a drop in volume. Our skin loses its bounce, feels drier and starts to sag. Our eyelids and the area around the mouth can also begin to slacken, pores become more visible and some women experience acne due to changes in hormone and sebum levels.

In your fifties: whether you're pre or postmenopausal, at this age collagen production declines by as much as 30 per cent. Along with the continued loss of elastin, a decrease in facial fat and bone shrinkage, means that our thinning skin succumbs to the pull of gravity. Our facial muscles weaken, dryness increases and lines become more prominent. The hot flushes that come part and parcel with the menopause can trigger or worsen rosacea, and our skin may become more sensitive. Age spots and pigmentation become more visible.

In your sixties and beyond: skin thinning can cause the face and neck to take on a crepey texture. You may have deeper lines around the mouth (nasolabial folds) and the eyes. Loss of fat volume and changes in bone structure in the middle face can make it appear sunken. Your eyelids may become hooded. You are likely to sweat less, but your skin is more prone to blotching, irritation and bruising.

The History of Massage

The beauty of massage is that it can go a long way to making our skin appear healthier and more youthful – without the use of knives or needles. Massage has a long history that dates back 5,000 years to India.[127] Passed down through the generations, massage has been used to relieve pain, heal injuries and prevent and cure various illnesses.

It became popular in China and South-East Asia, where it adopted practices from yoga, Chinese medicine and martial arts. Later, the Egyptians are credited with developing bodywork techniques that gave rise to reflexology. By 1868, a Dutch doctor named Johann Georg Mezger created what we now know as Swedish massage.[128] The list, of course, goes on and on!

Facial massage was included in these ancient therapies. However, it's thought that Western versions targeted toward cosmetic benefits are a more recent development. In both Europe and America, "facial fitness" has become something of a phenomenon. I love facial massage because it's a drug-free, non-invasive way to bring about a long list of benefits.

The benefits of focial massage include:

- Boosting circulation to give you an instant glow

- Stimulating lymphatic drainage to reduce puffiness

- Toning the muscles and re-contouring the face

- Accelerating detoxification

- Releasing muscular and facial tension, relieving headaches

- Helping your skincare products penetrate more effectively

- Softening facial lines

- Supporting scar tissue healing

- Easing sinus pressure and congestion

Depending on the type and technique, massage can also be energizing or calming. Even better, once you've found the right products and learned some techniques, home face massage is free. I like to do a quick massage in the morning to give my skin a rosy glow before applying make-up. Sometimes, I'll also do a massage in the evening while I'm watching TV to help prevent fluid accumulating overnight. It's also a great way to relax before you go to sleep.

Massage Glossary

These are some of the many methods I have been trained in and I can vouch for their benefits. Although many of these methods were originally designed for the body, I've adapted them to suit the muscles and tissues of the face.

Ayurvedic massage: based on the principles of Ayurveda (a Sanskrit word referring to "life" and "knowledge"), this treatment usually incorporates a lot of oil and also essential oils. Like other massage techniques, it relieves stress and muscular tension. However, Ayurvedic massage places more focus on the skin, using selected oils to nourish or rebalance it. Unlike other treatments that involve deep kneading motions, an Ayurvedic therapist may use a lighter, faster pressure with more rhythmic movements that stimulate circulation and bring about a deep sense of relaxation.

Facial reflexology: practised for centuries, this treatment relates to Traditional Chinese Medicine (TCM) and the belief that certain meridian points on our face correspond to organs within the body. By "mapping" the face and applying pressure to these points, practitioners aim to bring the body back into balance. Anecdotally, it's thought to help promote better sleep, relieve pain, increase energy levels, clear sinuses and elevate your mood.

Facial yoga: just as yoga keeps our bodies strong and pliable, so too facial yoga benefits our skin. Like a yoga class for the body, this holistic facial technique targets different muscle groups – and involves working inside your mouth, as well as on the external skin surface. Facial yoga targets the muscles that control our expressions, helping tone and strengthen the underlying skin structure. As you'd expect from a workout, facial yoga involves repeating these movements – and even pulsing – several times.

Indian face massage: the origins of this treatment are thought to lie with Kundan Mehta, a former schoolteacher who left India and arrived in London in the 1980s. Having trained in beauty therapy and a variety of different massage techniques, she combined Eastern and Western philosophies to devise a unique system of facial rejuvenation – what is now known as Indian face massage.[129] It involves gentle, repetitive movements that relieve tension, encourage mobility in stiffened tissue, tone the facial muscles, increase blood circulation and stimulate lymphatic drainage, leaving the skin looking lifted, refreshed and glowing.

Kobido massage: this treatment dates back to 15th century Japan,[130] and the name Kobido means "former path to beauty". Legend suggests that the samurais performed the technique after battles when they needed to restore calm and refocus their minds.[131] It's thought that the mix of fast and slow hand movements boost circulation and help promote collagen and elastin production.

Myofascial release: if you suffer from chronic headaches or back pain, fascia-based treatments might be a good one for you. Healthy, young fascia should be pliable and elastic, but over time, this matrix of connective tissue can become rigid. By stretching and massaging certain areas of the body with firm pressure, your therapist can help release this tightness in specific trigger points, causing pain. Releasing "sticky" fascia can often make us feel lighter and more energized. But be warned, the treatment itself is not always comfortable! There is often a burning sensation as the fascia is released.

Sports massage: although similar to deep tissue massage, a sports massage tends to target specific areas of the body. It analyses the impact of movement on the joints, muscles, tendons, ligaments and soft tissue. It's designed to support recovery from an injury or strain, enhance performance and encourage the removal of toxins (such as lactic acid) from the muscles. Sports massage incorporates a mix of stroking movements using the palms of the hands (effleurage), kneading (petrissage), rapid vibrations, deep tissue manipulation and working on pressure points along with friction-based motions that work on the muscles to support healing.

Swedish massage: works on the soft tissues and muscles while stimulating nerve endings and increasing blood flow and lymph drainage. It involves long strokes, kneading motions (petrissage), deep, circular movements and passive joint mobility. It's great if you tend to hold tension in your neck, shoulders or lower back – particularly after sitting at a desk all day. Deep tissue massage is very similar but uses a much firmer pressure to get into the muscles, tendons and fascia.

Thai massage: this stems from an ancient healing practice that uses deep pressure and stretching techniques to induce deep muscular release and relaxation. In some cases, your practitioner will ask you to participate in these movements. Thai massage is linked to reduced stress levels and increased energy. It also helps boost circulation, reduce headaches and improve joint mobility.

The Vodder Method: this is a Manual Lymphatic Drainage technique that I trained in early on in my career. It was developed in France in 1932 by doctors Emil and Estrid Vodder. While treating patients on the French Riviera, they noticed that many had swollen lymph nodes. This observation led them to develop the alternative medicine practice of "lymphology": the study of the lymphatic system.

The Vodder Method is an advanced massage technique that uses repetitive circular, spiral-shaped movements, which moves the skin over the underlying tissues using varying degrees of pressure. The change in pressure creates a pumping effect that encourages lymph flow, draining excess fluid from connective tissue.[132] Unlike blood, which relies on the heart to pump it around the body, the lymphatic system doesn't have its own pumping action, which is why we need to create it manually.

On the face, it helps reduce fluid retention and supports our cells' healing process. It also increases blood flow, delivering vital oxygen and nutrients to our skin, giving it an immediate lift and glow.

Massage Myth-busting

Massage is fantastic in many ways, but it will not eradicate lines and wrinkles. Neither will it reduce fat, help you lose weight on your face or make pigmentation vanish. It's also not a magic bullet. Just like a gym workout, you need to practice facial massage regularly if you want to reap the long-term benefits. And if you smoke or spend hours in the sun without applying SPF, then I'm afraid no amount of massage is going to counteract the damage to your skin.

Equally, don't be fooled into believing massage causes wrinkles (ageing, lifestyle factors and facial expressions do that). Applying pressure to the face won't stretch the skin or make it drop. I've been performing facial massage on clients for decades, as have many other practitioners around the world, and this has never been the case! By choosing the right products, using the right movements and applying the correct pressure, face massage will only benefit your skin.

The Best Products for Facial Massage

There are many different products you can use for a great facial massage. My preference is for plant-based oils, balms and cleansers. All of them have a viscous texture that supports the movement of your hands across your skin. There are many beautiful blended oils available on the market.

You need to use enough product to allow you to manipulate your face without tugging or dragging the skin. However, don't use so much that your fingers slip right off your face! Start with a small amount of product, and you can always add a little more if you feel any friction building up between your fingers and skin.

Some of my favourite oils for face massage (there are many more, of course!) are:

Coconut oil: wonderfully nourishing, it's ideal for dry skin and brings anti-inflammatory benefits.

Argan oil: rich in vitamin E, it helps heal and soothe inflammation.

Rosehip seed oil: light but packed full of vitamins, antioxidants and essential fatty acids, it also helps fade dark spots and supports scar healing.

Sea buckthorn oil: great for skin healing and regeneration, this is a good source of vitamins B and C, along with omegas 7 and 9.

Shea butter: more like a balm, so allows for a light texture and viscosity on the skin.

What not to use

Mineral oils and paraffin wax: both coat the skin and are likely to block pores, making them particularly disastrous for oily and acne-prone complexions.

Serums: being water-based, they tend to sink into the skin very quickly, rather than providing enough lubrication for massage. Save them for your regular skincare routine to ensure your skin gets a healthy kick of active ingredients, morning and night.

Moisturizers: again, these tend to absorb quickly, so are unsuitable for face massage, which can last anywhere between two and twenty minutes. Save them for adding extra hydration to your skin after applying your serum.

Aloe vera gel: while it's lovely and cooling, it quickly becomes tacky. Your fingers will probably get stuck to it!

My Massage No-no's

As transformative as facial massage can be, there are some circumstances that require us to take extra care.

If you have active acne: by all means, do a very gentle lymphatic drainage massage. However, anything more vigorous and stimulating should be avoided, as you'll only aggravate breakouts.

When suffering from rosacea: stimulating circulation will worsen the appearance of redness and visible blood vessels. Again, light lymphatic drainage is fine.

While applying prescription retinols: the dryness, flaking and sensitivity that comes with using prescription-strength retinol make it unsuitable for facial massage. Coming up a little pink is normal – and even a great sign that you've successfully encouraged healthy blood flow. However, sensitive skin can get very red and angry if massaged.

When you've been in the sun: hot and even slightly pink post-sun skin is only going to find massage irritating. Wait a few days until your skin is cooler and calmer.

If you're taking Roaccutane: this oral medication used to treat severe acne can cause the skin to thin, so take extra care not to tug the skin. Lymphatic drainage is, however, safe.

Using oil for lymphatic drainage: for all its popularity, it's amazing how many people still use an oil when they perform a lymphatic drainage massage. Using oil means you can easily slip past the delicate lymph nodes, meaning your massage may not be effective at all! Better to use clean, dry hands. As you're only making very light sweeping and pumping movements, you don't need the glide of an oil as you do with other massage techniques.

Your 101 on Massage Tools

In the same way that face massage has become increasingly popular, tools and gadgets are commonly used to support facial fitness.

Some facial massage tools create a nice sensation (and are particularly lovely when left to cool in the fridge or freezer). Others deliver real results when used consistently. You can perform a great face massage without them, so it's really a matter of personal preference.

These are some of the tools that I keep in my skincare kit:

Gua sha

In Chinese, *gua* means scraping and *sha* means disease. The treatment used by traditional Chinese medicine practitioners to treat the body has been adapted for cosmetic purposes on the face. You'll find that there's now an endless list of facial gua sha tools out there, made of materials such as rose quartz, amethyst, jade and stainless steel. They come in various shapes, often with curved edges that nestle into the facial contours to lift and sculpt them. They're great for lymphatic drainage and reducing puffiness. I always apply oil first. To get real results, you need to use yours regularly.

Jade and rose rollers

Like the gua sha, jade rollers are inspired by ancient Chinese tradition. They look a little like small paint rollers – and usually have one larger stone at the top for the forehead, cheeks, jaw and neck, and a smaller one at the bottom for around the eyes and chin. By rolling it back and forth over different areas of the face, using gentle pressure (and after applying oil), it's said to boost lymph flow and reduce puffiness. The Internet will often present jade rollers as a miracle anti-ageing tool and to be perfectly honest, this is not the case as results are limited. That said, jade rolling (especially if you keep yours in the fridge) can feel extremely soothing and always has a calming effect on my mind. These are valuable benefits in themselves – just don't expect your face to lose ten years after using one!

Cupping

You may well have heard about professional cupping treatments for the body in the media (they're popular among athletes and celebrities). The tradition is deeply ingrained in Chinese medicine and involves applying glass cups to the body. The cup is heated using a flame to create a suction effect that pulls blood into these areas, flooding the surrounding tissues with fresh, oxygenated blood while promoting new vessel formation. Cupping is also said to relieve muscle tension, support cell repair and encourage cell regeneration.

The treatment has more recently been used for rejuvenation purposes. Smaller, softer cups are used on the face, gently suctioning the skin away from the fascia and gliding across the face. I find that it's a great way to encourage lymph drainage, brighten the skin and encourage a lovely glow.

Spoons

An oldie but a goodie! One of the things I love about facial massage is that it's accessible to us all. So, if you don't want to spend money on tools, you can always pop two teaspoons in the freezer, ready for those mornings when you wake up to find your eyes looking tired and puffy. The cool sensation of the metal will help disperse the build-up of fluid, bring down that puffiness and make you feel more energized for your day ahead.

Facial Fitness FAQs

Once you've got the basis of facial anatomy and learned the key techniques detailed in the four-week plan, there's plenty of room for flexibility – so you can tailor your facial workouts according to your skin's needs, as well as the amount of time you have each day.

Just like physical movement, even a few minutes of facial massage can be beneficial. So, don't wait for a long window of time to squeeze it into your busy life – just do it as a matter of course, when you're cleansing your face, are applying oil at night, are watching TV or prepping your face for make-up. You can even do some quick lymphatic pumping movements while sitting at your desk throughout the day.

Here are some of the questions I get asked most when people start facial massage:

1. When should I massage?

Consistency is the most important thing here, so do your massage at whatever time works best for you. If morning works well, it's a great time to reduce any puffiness and boost your skin's glow before you apply make-up. If the evening is better, that's fine too.

2. Are there any times when I shouldn't massage?

Just as you would avoid a strenuous workout when suffering from a fever, virus or any illness that wipes you out energetically, this is a time when you can skip your facial massage and maximize rest. If you're receiving treatment for cancer, please seek advice from your specialist before trying any home massage methods.

3. Do I leave the oil on my skin after my massage?

Yes, you can do – especially if your skin is on the drier side and you don't plan to apply any other products afterwards. Alternatively, you can use a gentle wash to remove the oil then continue with your regular skincare routine.

4. Can I apply my serum over the oil?

Not really. The oil will create a barrier that prevents the active ingredients within your serum from penetrating the skin effectively. So, wash the oil off, then apply your serum.

5. Why am I breaking out after my massage?

You could be using an oil that's too rich for your skin type. See page 109 for the oils I recommend for oil- or blemish-prone skin. You should also ensure that you wash off excess oil after massaging and may want to reduce the number of facial workouts you do per week.

6. Should my massage feel painful?

In certain areas where we hold a lot of tension, such as the jaw and neck, massage can feel a little uncomfortable. You might feel tightness followed by the easing of "knotty" areas. However, you should never feel sharp or severe pain.

7. I can feel bobbly lumps when I massage. Is this normal?

Yes! The underlying skin structures and fat can sometimes feel a little odd and knobbly. If you're coming down with something or are fighting off a virus, you might also feel the lymph nodes in your neck move, like small pearls, beneath the skin. If you notice something new that persists for a few days, I'd always suggest getting it checked out by your doctor.

8. How often can I do facial massage?

It's really up to you. You might choose to do some movements every day, performing them as you cleanse your skin, perhaps. The weekly plan includes plenty of techniques to help you target different facial areas and skin needs. If your skin becomes sensitive, reduce the length of each massage and cut back on the number of times you're doing it each week. And if you're under the age of twenty, three times a week is more than enough.

9. How long before I see results?

We're all different, so results vary from person to person. You might see some immediate benefits; even just one massage can temporarily reduce puffiness around your eyes, make your cheeks appear more lifted and leave your skin fresh and glowing. With regular facial workouts, you'll begin to see more lasting results.

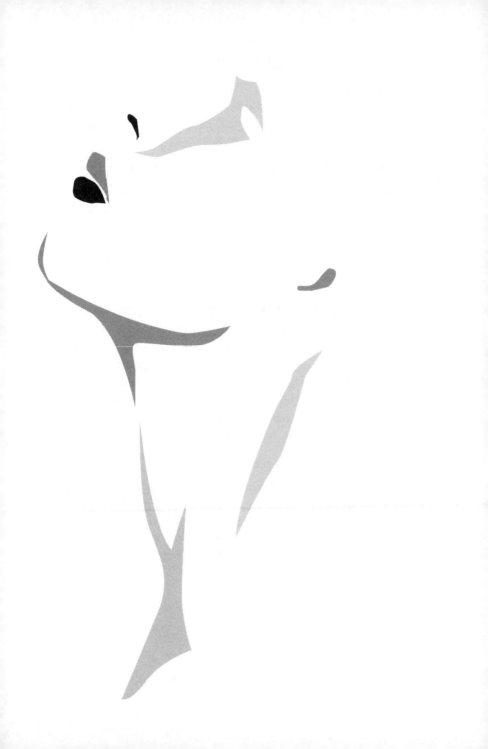

8

How Does the Glow Plan Work?

In chapters 1 to 7, we delved into many internal and external factors that impact your skin's health and vitality. By introducing facial massage, as well as making some lifestyle changes that support our mental and physical wellness, we can make a real improvement to how we look and feel.

Health benefits:

- Better circulation
- Relieves muscle tension
- Supports the lymphatic system

Emotional benefits:

- Greater confidence
- Happiness

- Energy

- Feeling calm

Physical benefits:

- Skin radiance

- More defined facial contours

- Reduces puffiness

- A more youthful-looking complexion

Using the Plan

Firstly, it's important to say that the plan sets out some guidelines. Nothing is set in stone, but the closer you follow them, the better the results. We all know the more we put in, the more we get out. But this isn't supposed to be punishment – it's about setting yourself up to age well. Humans are creatures of habit and making changes can be challenging, frustrating and feel clunky. So, don't worry if there are aspects of the plan that feel difficult. That's OK! Focus on what comes more naturally – then work through anything that feels trickier.

The Glow Plan does not set goals, because different people will get different results. If the outcome is that you have more energy, feel happier, and have enjoyed the process or learnt something new, that's a huge win. If your skin is more glowy, you're getting compliments from friends and family and your facial contours are more defined, then that's even better!

Each week we'll be expanding your knowledge and building on your skillset by focusing on a key lifestyle theme – and a target area for your skin.

Things to remember:

- You're investing this time in yourself

- Week 1 can feel exciting as you learn new things; by week 3, it can be challenging to maintain momentum. Be kind to yourself and keep going

- Set yourself some time each day. There are 1,440 minutes in a day. I believe that *everyone* can find at least five to ten of these for themselves!

- As a general rule repeat every move five to ten times

Non-negotiables:

- Do the warm-ups

- Move your body to positively impact your face. They are connected, after all!

- Practise cold water splashing

- Target problem areas

- Turn to the quick-fix moves when you're short on time

FAQs

1. When should I start?

NOW!

2. What if I have Botox or fillers?

Wait two weeks after Botox and six weeks after fillers before starting any of the massage techniques. You can start all other aspects of the plan right away.

3. Do I have to massage my face daily?

Aim for a minimum of five minutes a day. Once this becomes a natural part of your life, you won't even realize you're doing it.

4. My face comes up pink after massaging. Is that normal?

Yes, because we're actively stimulating blood flow, which gives us a rosy glow. That said, everyone's skin responds differently. As women, our skin can also change throughout our monthly cycle. If you're very red, consider using less pressure or a different oil. Have a look at the skincare section to see my recommendations for sensitive skin. On some days, you may simply want to perform the very light lymphatic moves.

5. Is it better to do five minutes a day or twenty minutes once a week?

My preference is regular daily practice. Let's say a minimum of five days a week.

6. What's the best time of day to perform massage?

There's no right or wrong here, so find what works for you. I'll also give you some guidelines for morning and evening routines.

7. Am I too young?

No. However, under the age of twenty-five, your skin and body is still regenerating well. You don't need to massage your face daily.

8. Am I too old?

Absolutely not! It's never too late to start feeling great.

Do:

- Start by practising your massage techniques in front of a mirror, so you can see where you're working and be more precise with your movements.

- Repeat your massage on both sides of your face, unless you're targeting facial asymmetry.

- For lifting massage, always create slip by using an oil, balm or cleansing cream.

- For lymphatic massage, use dry, clean hands – no product.

- Enjoy! You're investing time in something that's special, so make sure you have fun.

Don't:

- Press so hard that it hurts. Some moves can feel uncomfortable, especially when we are working on fascial release. But you shouldn't be in agony.

- Use serums or mineral oils (we covered this in Chapter 6).

- Hold your breath while massaging. Instead, think about lowering your shoulders and feeling more relaxed.

- Just focus on one routine or movement that you find easy. Mix it up and give your face the full benefits of combined methods.

Getting started

The only equipment for the exercises in this book is:

- A gua sha (or spoon)

- A mirror

- Cleanser

- A massage medium, ideally an oil or balm

- A hair band

- A damp cloth for cleansing and removing excess oil

- A willingness to invest this time in yourself

Let's start by taking photos of your face. Make sure you remove your make-up, tie your hair back and find somewhere with natural lighting. Take your photos:

- Straight on

- From the left-hand side

- From the right-hand side

These images are just for your reference to help you track progress. We don't often see our faces from different angles and it's good to have a starting point.

(If you want to share some "before and afters" with me, I would love to see them on Instagram!)

It can take anywhere from 18 to 254 days for a person to form a new habit and an average of 66 days for a new behaviour to become automatic. There's no one-size-fits-all, which is why the time frame is so broad; some habits are also easier to form than others and we are all so individual.

Each week we'll be working on both physical and emotional habits under a specific theme.

You have the knowledge from the first half of this book, so now it's up to you!

For every week of the Glow Plan you'll find:

1. **Affirmations:** these are best done in the morning. I've made some suggestions, but go with what feels right for you. If you can say them out loud to yourself, even better. Then repeat the affirmation to yourself throughout the day.

2. **Gratitude:** make it a daily habit to remember the things you're thankful for. Being grateful is one of the simplest things we can do, and yet it's so immensely powerful. We have the power to recondition the mind. Over time this will become an unconscious process.

3. **Happiness:** I know that this is sometimes easier said than done, but a happy face is a beautiful face and smiling is contagious! We're going to keep it simple and each week list three things that make you happy.

4. **A breathing technique:** these will vary depending on the focus of the week. Some will be better suited to the evening, others can be carried out at any time throughout the day.

5. **Physical activity:** this will vary in intensity. Where possible, there are some modifications given to suit all levels. Do also continue with any other activities and sports you already enjoy!

6. **Physical support:** methods to support the body's natural elimination processes (don't worry, there are no enemas!) and overall health.

7. **Vitamin N (Nature):** it might sound odd to recommend going outside as a means of improving your skin. But check back in with what we covered in Chapter 3 and you'll see why.

8. **Nutrition:** each week, you'll discover nutritional tips, including foods to add in and foods to ditch.

9. **Skincare:** we'll be removing some things and replacing them with others to build a routine that better supports your skin.

10. **Meditation:** this will vary from week to week, always with the aim of enhancing your mental and emotional wellbeing. Even if you start with one minute a day, it's better to achieve small steps than nothing at all.

11. **Face massage:** we'll cover daily routines, along with deep dives into supporting specific areas of your face and specialized techniques for certain skin concerns.

12. **Journalling:** whether you make notes in this book or somewhere else, journalling is an important part of the process and I encourage you to do it daily. However, if you miss a day, don't worry – just begin again the next day.

> "The more you count your blssings, the more blessings you will have to count."
> – (traditional saying)

For those with acne or rosacea, some of the lifting massage techniques won't be suitable for your skin. For specific massage that that's more beneficial for your skin type, see the lymphatic massage in week 2.

Have fun and enjoy the process!

Progress not perfection!

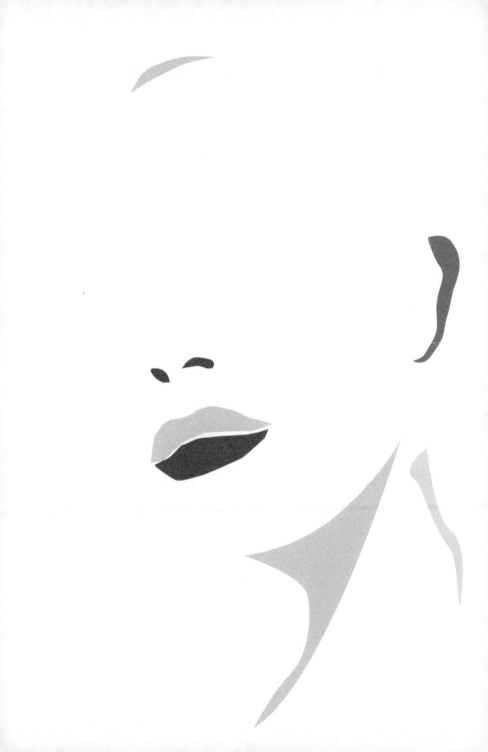

9

The Glow Plan: Week 1

Changing your Mindset and Massage Basics

Focus area: neck and chest

This week is about establishing the basics and forming new patterns. As in all aspects of your life, mindset is fundamental to succeed with this plan. Let's use this week to mentally prepare yourself for change and growth. It's perfectly natural to find this week challenging, as there are many new things to try. You may also find it extremely fulfilling and exciting as you set out on your path to ageing well.

Let's get going!

Gratitude

My life is a gift; I am lucky to be here.
I am thankful for my unique creativity and mind.

Happiness

Today I choose to be happy.

Things to remember:

- Success starts in the mind

- Self-improvement is hard work

- Consistently working on your mindset every day is the secret to health and happiness

- Good mental health is timeless

- If you don't make change, you can't expect change to happen

- It doesn't matter what other people think of you. What's important is what you think of yourself

- Progress, not perfection

- Focus on *why* you're doing this, not how you're going to do it

- Be intentional with your time. Block time to be on your phone rather than being on your phone all the time.

Four weeks from now, you're going to look and feel more radiant – and may even have taken a few years off your perceived age. Don't underestimate the power of consistency: it's essential that you dedicate time every day to taking action for your short- and long-term benefit. Stop doubting yourself! Harness your power and know that you're worth it; you deserve to age well – inside and out.

Many of us are highly critical of what we see in the mirror. Try not to compare yourself to others, and don't believe everything you see on social media: it's easy for someone to share glossy images and fabulous words about living their best life. Don't compare your behind-the-scenes with someone else's final performance. Instead of thinking about what everyone else is doing, focus on *you*.

Affirmations

I am confident, beautiful and strong.
I can and I will.
I don't have to be perfect to be confident.
I am powerful, I am capable.

Breathwork

5-3-8 breath

This method is something I've used for years, and have even taught to my children. It's a simple yet effective way of regaining control over your breathing patterns.

   The aim here is to inhale and exhale fully. As if by magic, it makes you feel both calm and re-energized. Little and often is key, so start with two to five minutes each day and increase to as much time as feels good.

1. Sit or lie somewhere comfortable. Close your eyes (if you're on a bus or somewhere public, don't feel the need to close your eyes – focus on the process of breathing).

2. Drop your shoulders and soften your jaw.

3. Inhale through your nose for a slow count of five (just as we did at school when playing hide and seek: think one elephant, two elephants …). Feel your chest expand. Hold the breath at the top for the count of three.

4. Slowly breathe out through your nose for the count of eight, fully emptying your lungs, right to the bottom.

5. Repeat for eight or more rounds, making each transition flow into the next breath to create full, rounded breathing. Then let your breath return to a normal pattern.

Nutrition

This week we'll have a clear-out to set some key markers for better health and long-term success. If you have any underlying health issues, are pregnant or breastfeeding, please take advice from your specialist before making any dramatic changes to your diet.

Remove sugar, including sweets, cakes, biscuits, fizzy drinks containing refined sugar, maple syrup, honey and sugar alternatives If your reaction is "no way!", review Chapter 5 on gut health to remind yourself why you're doing this.

Here are some replacements for when you're craving that sweet fix. It's worth noting that while fruit does contain sugar, it's also packed full of free-radical-fighting antioxidants.

> **Banana:** baked bananas, banana chips
> **Stewed apple:** with the skin removed as some people are allergic to it
> **Pear/mango/grapes/dates/blueberries** (it's amazing how quickly a punnet can be devoured!)
> **Dark chocolate:** 60 per cent cocoa solids or higher

Aim to remove saturated fats, processed meat, junk food – burgers, pizza, kebabs, nachos, fried chicken, chips.

Add in healthy oils such as avocados, nuts, olive oil, sunflower seeds, pumpkin seeds. Plus greens, such as broccoli, cabbage, lettuce, sprouts, green beans, kale, spinach, celery, cucumber.

Hydration

I recommend getting a reusable water bottle. The popular metal ones are usually around 500ml, or just under a pint. You should aim for three to four pints of water per day. Having a bottle that holds a pint makes it easy to track your intake, as you know that you need to refill it three or four times a day.

Herbal teas do count, as does hot water with any additions like lemon or ginger. Black tea and coffee *don't* count – and neither does alcohol!

Vitamin N: Get Outside

This week, get outside and walk – every day – for at least twenty minutes. This might sound simple, but it can be a challenge. Prepare for the weather and dress appropriately, and just get outside. If it's hot, apply your SPF, wear loose clothing and walk early in the morning or evening when the sun is cooler. Walking is free and easily accessible. Walk with purpose and make sure your get your daily step count in. You're aiming for 8–10,000 a day.

While you're outside, look around and take in your surroundings. Take time to notice the trees, buildings and other people that pass by. Don't forget to look up – especially at night-time, when you might be lucky enough to enjoy starry skies.

Whenever you need to go somewhere, ask yourself: "Could I walk there?" Or even, "Could I walk *part* of the way?" Many of us have gotten into the habit of driving, or getting an Uber or bus. But if the answer to either question is "yes", then walk.

Dry Body Brushing

Aim to practise dry body brushing every day, before showering or bathing. Brushing stimulates blood flow and the lymphatic system while exfoliating the skin, and generally gives you a wake-up call.

You'll need:

- **A dry body brush**

- **5–8 minutes**

1. Start on the upper thigh area, focusing on one leg at a time. Brush using circular movements, working inward and upward, going over the same area three to five times. Continue until you've covered the entire upper thigh –

front, back and middle. Don't forget your bottom! Follow this with long, sweeping upward strokes over your thighs.

2. Do the same on the lower leg, using small circular motions. Then make big, upward circles over the whole lower leg, moving around the ankle, up to the knee, then from the knee to the groin. Repeat on the other leg.

3. Circle the brush over your abdomen, using big circular movements. Move from your right to your left side.

4. Brush your arms, working from your hands and wrists to your elbows, using smaller circular movements. Then sweep upward from your elbow to your shoulder, on the front and back of the arm. Repeat on the other arm.

5. Sweep from shoulder to shoulder from left to right, then brush downward from your neck to your chest.

6. Brush your back using the same circular motions, covering as much as you can reach.

Physical Activity

Let's get going with some stretches for the body. We'll start gently and build up to something more vigorous. The best time to perform your morning stretches is just before your daily facial massage. The muscles and tissues of our face and neck are connected to those of our head and the rest of our body.

These simple stretches will form part of your every-morning routine. Hold each stretch or position for the count of five to eight seconds, or longer.

Sit or stand in an upright position. Shrug your shoulders down, away from your ears, letting your arms hang loosely by your sides.

Stretch 1

Move your left ear over to your left shoulder, feel the stretch down the right side of your neck. Rest your left hand on the right-hand side of your head, gently increasing the stretch. You can also deepen the stretch by reaching your right hand down toward the floor. Repeat on the other side.

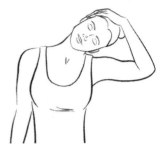

Stretch 2

Keep your back straight to create a stretch in the front of your neck and décolleté. Place your fingers on your collarbone and add some downward tension to increase the stretch. Closing your jaw will deepen the sensation further. Press your tongue onto the roof of your mouth using a repetitive pumping action, pursing your lips at the same time.

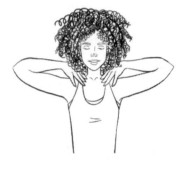

Stretch 3

Clasp your hands behind your head and look down. Use your hands to apply a little pressure and feel the stretch run down the back of your neck. Don't pull so hard that it's painful. You should feel a nice release.

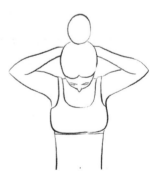

Stretch 4

Move your head in a semi-circle. Start at one ear, arc down so you're looking at the floor, then move back up to the other side. Repeat in the opposite direction.

Stretch 5

Place your hands on your shoulders. Rotate your elbows forward and back, creating large circles. Allow your chest to open. Do five rotations backward, then five forward.

Stretch 6A

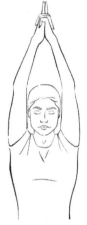

Raise your arms above your head with your hands in prayer position. Release your index fingers. Then stretch up toward the ceiling, letting your shoulders slide downward. Enjoy the feeling of length in your body as you grow taller, keeping your arms close to your ears.

Stretch 6B

Holding your core tight, side bend over to the right to feel the length open up all down your ribs and left-hand side. Hold for a count of five, return to centre, then repeat on the other side.

Stretch 7

Clasp your hands behind your back with your arms straight to open your chest. If you can't clasp your hands behind your back, place your hands on your lower back as far you can. Squeeze your upper back together, then look up and lean backward. Lower your head to its regular position. Then fold forward – your clasped hands will begin to move over your head. Let your chest rest on your thighs in this forward fold for five deep breaths.

Stretch 8

From your forward fold, release your arms and hands to the floor. Rock your body from left to right, clasping each elbow with the opposite hand in a ragdoll position. Let your head hang heavy, nod "yes" and shake "no". Keep your knees as bent as you need to, so as not to pull on your hamstrings or lower back.

Stretch 9

Come into a forward fold with your knees slightly bent again, and your feet hip-distance apart. Place your right hand on the floor as you rotate

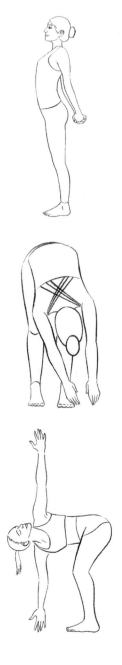

toward the left, lifting your left hand up to the ceiling. Let your head follow the arc of your hand, but don't strain your neck.

Windmill your left arm down to meet your right and place it on the floor. Repeat the last movement on the other side, this time twisting toward the right as your right hand and gaze move upward.

Place both hands on the floor and slowly roll up the spine, one vertebra at a time, until you're standing up straight.

Stretch 10

Give yourself a big hug as you wrap your arms around your body, placing each hand on the opposite shoulder blade. Keep your hips facing straight forward. Release your arms and perform the same stretch, this time placing the opposite arm on top.

Skincare

Week 1 is all about making a few simple but important changes.

Remove:

- Perfumed skincare products

- Any products you suspect aren't really working

- Physical exfoliants and weekly masks

- Anything with "SLS" on the ingredient list (see page 72)

Your morning routine

Step 1: Massage

Before cleansing (this is key!) massage your face with oil for three to five minutes. Then cleanse.

Step 2: Cleanse

Cleanse every morning, using something gentle but effective, such as a cream wash. Set a timer on your phone for one minute. Cleansers need about a minute to work, so let's allow your skin the time it needs to thrive. Use a warm or hot cloth to remove your cleanser.

Step 3: Cool

As part of our daily skincare practice, you're going to cold-water cleanse. Splash your face and neck with cold water a minimum of ten times. If you want to avoid getting your hair wet, you can always wear a shower cap or headband. Alternatively, create a cold compress using a flannel and hold it onto your face and neck for ten seconds each. Rinse and repeat three times. If you want to add some ice cubes to a bowl of water that's great.

Step 4: Tonic

This is optional. But, as we're not using any harsh acids within your morning routine this week, a hydrating tonic can be a nice addition.

Step 5: Serum

Something hydrating and/or with antioxidants.

Step 6: Moisturizer

A day cream that's suitable for your skin.

Step 7: Eye cream

If you're over the age of thirty.

Step 8: Sunscreen

No lower than SPF 30.

Home gadgets (optional)

LED face masks: can be used two to four times a week, morning or evening. They're safe for all skin types but should not be used during pregnancy.

Deep Dive: Facial Muscles

The muscles responsible for our facial expressions are hugely important, as they act as a means of non-verbal communication. They're unique in the fact that they generally originate from the skull. Unlike most skeletal muscles, which insert into another bone, the muscles of the face are attached to the superficial fascia, dermis of the skin, or even other muscles. When they contract, the skin moves, forming facial expressions – all without us even having to think about it!

Each muscle has an origin and insertion point – or the area where it starts and finishes. These points are where the muscle attaches to another structure. The muscles involved in chewing (such as the outer jaw, masseter and temple-area temporalis) are connected to bone at each end. All other facial muscles are attached from bone to tissue.

Interestingly, when our facial muscles contract, they move the skin rather than the joint, as other muscles within the body do. Imagine lifting a bag: when your bicep muscle contracts, your arm moves. But when facial muscles contract and move, they create expression lines in the skin.

···· Face Massage ····

This week, we're establishing a daily massage practice for face and upper body. It only takes three to five minutes, and it'll form the foundation of your routine going forward.

First, we'll massage without oil, working on the muscles which are connected bone to bone. These are the stronger muscles that hold more tension.

The temples, occipital and outer jaw (no oil)

1. Your hair can be loose or tied back. Firmly place your fingers on your outer jaw in front of your ears. Creating small, firm, circular motions, massage this area, keeping your fingers together as you open and close your mouth. This will help release the jaw muscles. Repeat this, massaging in the opposite direction..

2. On the temples in front of and above your ears, make firm circular forward motions that move the tissue, rather than just gliding over the skin. Massage around this whole area, circling forward then backward five times in each direction.

3. Place your fingers at the base of your skull. At the top of your neck, perform circular massage movements, using a firm pressure as you work from the base of your skull out toward your ears. Firmly place your fingers either side of the spine on your neck. Pull your fingers forward squeezing toward your palms, creating a nice deep massage move.

4. Firmly clasp your upper trapezius with your palms on the sides of your neck. Stretch your neck from side to side without rotating it. Use the pressure of your hand to create a stretch down each side of your neck. You might feel heat within the skin as you create friction and increase blood flow. This is perfectly normal!

FACE MASSAGE

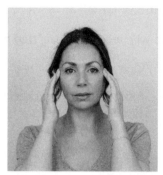

2.

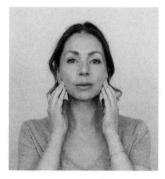

1a.

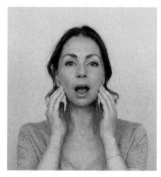

1b.

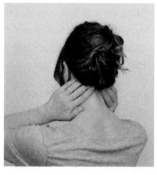

3.

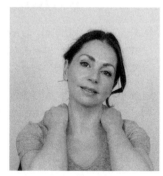

4.

Start with oil

You will need your hair tied back:

1. Apply oil to the palms of your hands.

2. Smooth it over your cheeks, forehead, chin and neck, working from the middle of your face, outward and down.

···· Neck massage release ····

1. Starting on the neck, place your right hand on the left-hand side of your lower neck to support the skin. Use the other hand to massage the skin, using downward circles, followed by firm upward glides. Switch sides.

2. For the middle section of your neck, use a lighter pressure, gliding one hand up and off at the chin, with your hand in a cupping motion.

···· Glide-out prayers ····

1. Put your hands in prayer position, with your thumbs underneath your jaw. Glide outward, pushing across your face from nose to ear.

2. Using the palms of your hands, push both cheeks up at the same time, moving from your jaw to your cheekbones.

NECK MASSAGE RELEASE

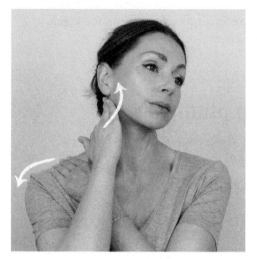

GLIDE-OUT PRAYERS

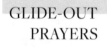

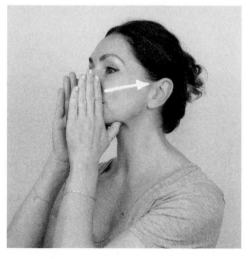

•••• V push-ups ••••

1. Create a V with your index and middle finger and push your nasolabial line and cheeks upward. Squish your fingers together so they join just in front of your ear, then glide back down your face. Repeat five times.

•••• Lip plumper ••••

1. Using your middle and index fingers and a firm pressure, sweep around your entire mouth and lip area.

2. Purse your lips as you create small, tight circles with your fingers.

•••• Under-eye glides ••••

1. Using your index and middle fingers, glide in an outward direction, working beneath your eyes. Move from the side of your nose to the sides of your face. Repeat five times.

2. Circle the eyes with your middle finger, pushing up under the brow as you glide outward. Trace back underneath the eye, but don't drag the skin. Repeat this movement with a bigger circle, going above the brow.

•••• Frown line eraser ••••

1. Using your middle fingers, move up and down from the brow to the hair line. Repeat this movement, working

V PUSH-UPS

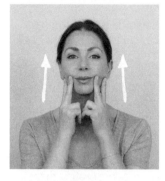

LIP PLUMPER

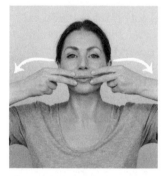

1.

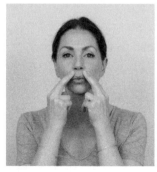

2.

UNDER-EYE GLIDES

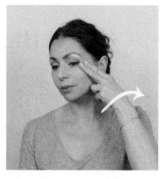

1.

FROWN LINE ERASER

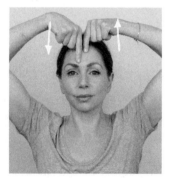

1.

outward to the sides of your face so you cover the entire forehead. Circle under the eyes and repeat this three times.

2. Smooth down over the face, gliding down the side of the neck

3. Wash off your oil with a gentle cleanser

✦ Gadget Highlight: Teaspoons ✦

Teaspoons are easily accessible and simple to use. You can start with using one, then try two at the same time. When incorporating them into your massage routine, make sure you apply oil to your skin first. Place your index finger in the middle of the dip of the spoon to help guide it.

1. Support the skin at the chin with the hand not holding the teaspoon. Create a rocking movement with the curve of the spoon on the skin and caterpillar outward across the jaw and cheeks.

2. Glide the teaspoon from your chin, across the jaw to your ear three times.

3. Support the sides of the mouth and repeat this movement further up, working across your cheek to your ear.

4. Support the side of your nose and repeat, moving under your eyes to your temples.

5. Glide up and out under your brow.

6. Glide out from middle of your forehead to the side in two to three horizontal lines.

7. Glide down the sides of your neck.

8. Repeat on the other side of your face.

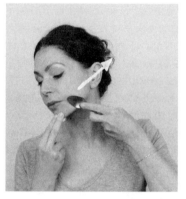

1.

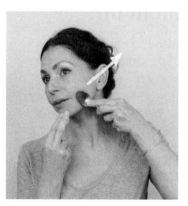

2.

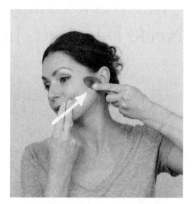

3.

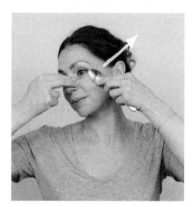

4.

This Week's Target Area: Neck/Décolleté/Jawline

Your neck has the important job of holding your head up, and we tend to hold a lot of tension in our necks. The skin is generally more delicate than on the face; our décolleté has less fat beneath the skin surface, so is also finer. We may see a lot of sun damage in this area. The muscles here are not necessarily involved in forming facial expressions, but the state of our neck has a huge impact on our overall appearance and vitality of our skin. For these reasons, working on the neck fascia is vital. It's essential that we respect the lymphatic system and key lymph nodes (see page 127–8).

When performing fascial release, we always start by easing the largest muscles. This allows other, smaller muscles to relax too. As we discovered in Chapter 7, fascia is immensely strong, and this strength means that some of these moves might be uncomfortable, and you may even feel a slight burning sensation. Don't worry – this is a sign it's working!

···· Fascial neck and décolleté ···· release – without oil

1. For your trapezius: Place one hand on your opposite shoulder. Pinch and hold your traps, close to your neck (I find lifting the shoulders allows you to grab hold of the muscle). Hold this position for ten seconds. Relax your shoulders and breathe. Release, pinch and lift slightly further out. Repeat on the other side.

2. Place your knuckles under your occipital bone (at the base of your skull), push in firmly and hold. Bend your head backward (look up) to deepen the sensation. Firmly and

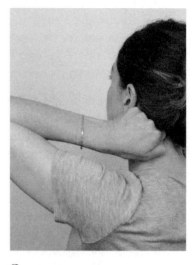

2.

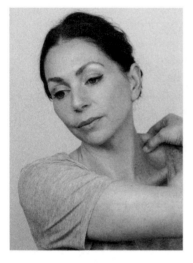

1.

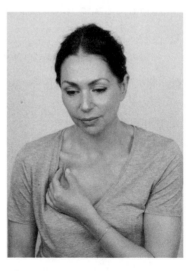

4.

slowly, glide your knuckles down the back of your neck. Rock your knuckles into the muscles if you find they're not able to glide easily over your skin. This feeling is right on the boundary between pleasure and pain! Repeat on the other side. As a side note, this technique is great for easing migraines.

3. Put one hand on the opposite side of your neck and bend your head forward. Starting under your ear, pinch and hold in two to three places as you move down the muscle. Repeat on the other side.

4. At the middle of your décolleté, just under the clavicle, use your thumbs and forefingers to pinch and hold the tissue as you roll your shoulders forward to release muscular tension. Relax your shoulders back. Slowly roll (almost feels like folding over) the skin from the midline outward. Repeat, working outward in the same manner across one side of your décolleté toward your armpit (do this two to three times), then do the other side. You will feel heat in the tissue and some redness.

5. Use your fingers to press firmly at the clavicle. Move outward, pressing and holding.

6. Tap across the whole area of the décolleté, neck and shoulders.

Neck and jawline massage with oil

Apply oil to the area and repeat each movement three to eight times.

1. Make a scissor motion at either side of your ears, using your index and middle fingers.

2. Use the same fingers to circle behind your ears, using a firm pressure.

3. Look up slightly, creating space between your chin and your chest. Place both hands under your jaw with the sides of your pointing fingers on your skin one in front of the other. Pull the hands apart and together, creating a friction with the sides of your fingers with the skin under your jaw. Move back and forth covering the whole area under the jaw.

4. Place your knuckles under your jaw and glide out toward your ear. Repeat on the other side.

5. Repeat, using both knuckles to sweep along each side of the jaw at the same time.

6. With your knuckle and thumb pushing out under your jaw, pinch and glide out from your chin to your ears (both hands at the same time). Repeat this move until you've covered your entire neck.

7. Support your neck with one hand and use the fingers of your other hand to create flicking movements up one side of the neck. Start with two fingers, then use all four. Repeat on the other side of the neck.

8. Place the palm of your hand under your chin and push up beneath your jaw as you glide outward toward your ear. Repeat on the other side, then do it again using both hands at the same time.

NECK AND JAWLINE MASSAGE WITH OIL

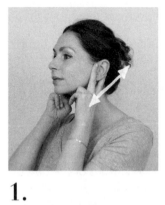

1.

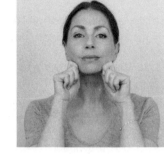

6.

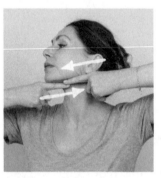

3.

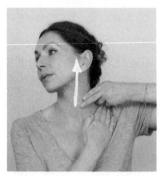

7a.

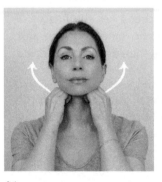

5.

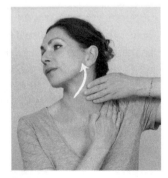

7b.

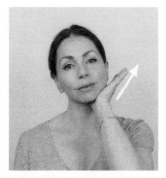

8a.

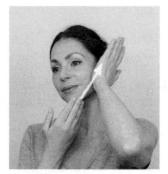

12.

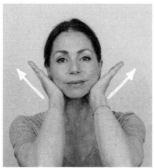

8b.

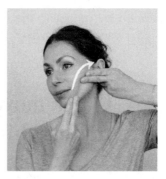

13.

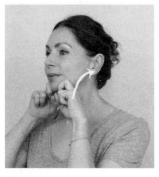

9.

9. With the knuckles of your middle and forefinger, spread like folded bunny ears, under and above your jawline, glide out from chin to ear.

10. Use the same knuckle motion on one side of your face, using one thumb to push outward from chin to ear.

11. Use the pads on the palms of your hands to push outward from chin to ear, just above the jaw.

12. Place your palm on one side of your face. Lift and hold for a count of ten and repeat on the other side.

13. Support your jaw with one hand. Use two fingers from the other hand to flick upward, working along the jawline.

14. Finish by repeating the scissoring motion either side of your ears before gliding downward.

···· Quick moves to support a ···· double chin – without oil

A double chin, also known as submental fat, is a common condition that occurs when a layer of fat forms below your chin. It's often associated with weight gain, but you don't have to be overweight to have one. Genetics or looser skin that occurs as a result of ageing may also be the cause. Face massage won't get rid of fat, but it can help support the skin by firming the muscles and draining fluid.

1. A face yoga move: place your fingers on your clavicle. Hold the skin with your fingertips as you look up and feel a stretch. Open and close your jaw five times. Place your tongue on the roof of your mouth while pursing your lips. Repeat the whole process ten times.

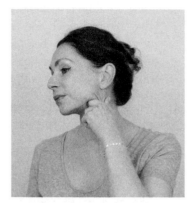

2b.

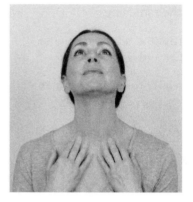

1.

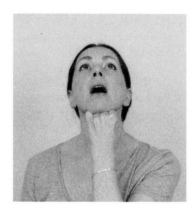

5.

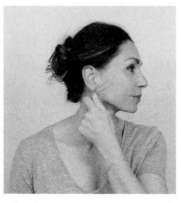

2a.

2. Using the thumb and knuckle of your forefinger: start under your chin and pinch and twist, moving your knuckle toward the thumb as you work toward your ear. Glide your fingers down your neck and repeat on the other side. Remember to support your skin with the other hand as you do this.

3. Repeat the same movement, but this time use both hands, working out toward each ear at the same time.

4. Make small pinching motions across the whole chin area, starting at the middle and working outward.

5. Place your fist beneath your chin and push upward. Open and close your mouth using your fist as resistance.

6. Tilt your head back and look up to the sky. Place both thumbs under your chin and glide outward. Push your tongue into the roof of your mouth. Repeat.

Myofascial release

This method is usually performed without oil, so it's easier to grab hold of the tissue, skin and muscle. Perform a pinching movement and move across the underlying structure slowly to allow the fascia to release.

A 5-minute Meditation

Let's take this one step further, using the same breathing pattern as we did before. Imagine releasing stress and tension every time you exhale. Breathe out anything negative that pops into your mind. It could be heat, a colour, an emotion or feeling.

With each inhale, imagine something positive: a bright colour, flowers, a rainbow – whatever comes to mind. Stick with the item you've chosen rather than switching between different ones. This helps give you something to focus on as you reap the powerful benefits of deep breathing. Remember: inhale the good, exhale the bad.

It's helpful to focus on something – rather than empty space. When thoughts enter your mind, acknowledge them and let them pass. Then return your focus to the present moment. If you can accept that continuously bringing your mind back to the present moment is the meditation, it will be much easier to keep your mind still, rather than getting frustrated.

Journalling

This week, I want to focus on making journalling a part of your daily life. Find a time that works for you and stick to it. You can write free flow; just get your thoughts, emotions and anything that cropped up in your day down on paper.

Some things to cover:

- How are you feeling on a scale. of one to five? (one being bad, five being amazing)

- How do you feel about your skin and ageing?

- Write down your main concerns

- Write down three things you love about your face and or body

- What are your energy levels like today?

- If it's the beginning of the week, how are you feeling about the week ahead?

- At the end of the week: how are you feeling about the last few days? Were there any significant high or low points?

Congratulations on completing Week 1!

Some space for your thoughts

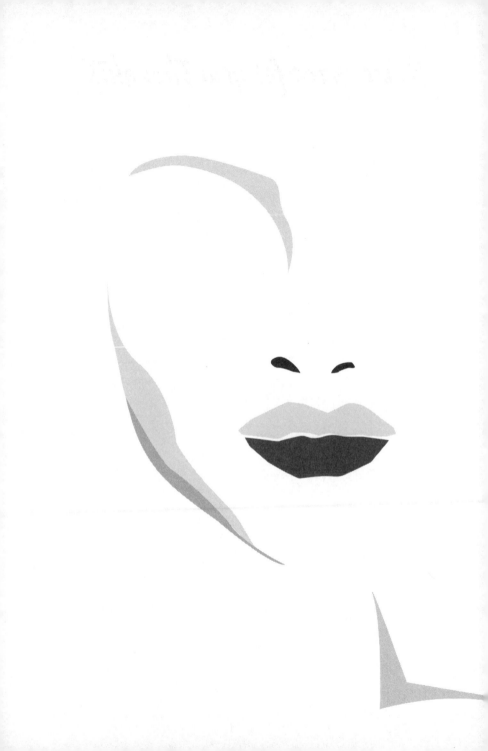

10

The Glow Plan: Week 2

Sleep Well to Age Well

Focus area: jawline/cheeks, lymphatics, skin needling

The theme of this week is sleep. As you move through this week, look back at Chapter 2 for more hints and tips to optimize your sleep. Good-quality sleep is essential to our wellbeing and the vibrancy of our skin. I've dedicated this whole week to supporting a good night's rest, while continuing to build on the habits we began in Week 1.

The objective of this week's focus is to become more aware of your sleep cycle and make any adjustments. Many of us struggle for days, weeks, months – years – with poor-quality sleep. Now's the time to notice what's happening – then create new habits that change things for the better.

What you'll need this week for better sleep: Your bed, a soft pillow and socks for keeping your feet warm if it's cold.

Gratitude

Practising gratitude has been proven to be hugely helpful for those with sleep issues. If I can't sleep, I often find going through a mental list of things and people in my life that I'm grateful for is a brilliant way to calm the mind.

This week I am thankful for …
I'm grateful for <name/place/thing> in my life because …
Something that I take for granted is <fill in>, but I am grateful for this because …

———————

Happiness

List three things that have made you happy this week.

———————

Affirmations

I am calm and confident in every situation
I choose to be kind to myself
My self-care is a priority
Stress and worry do not control me; I choose to remain calm
and grounded.

On the next page you'll find some specific affirmations for the evening, which work a bit like self-hypnosis or autosuggestion – a technique that was developed by an apothecary at the beginning of the 20th century as a means of guiding our own thoughts.

In the past, I've benefited from hypnotherapy. I still use some of the words and visualisations I learnt in my first session twenty-five years ago, which I attended out of a need to get my emotions back under control and regain a sense of calm.

One visualisation I remember particularly vividly is a walking journey through a gate at the end of a garden. Down some steps; a secret beach; feeling the sand beneath my toes. Then the sound of the waves, finding shells on the beach and the smell of the sea.

The thing that links all these techniques together is that they help us change our internal narrative. So, instead of tossing and turning, and worrying about why you can't sleep and how tired you'll be in the morning, you create a new story for yourself. Almost like a script for good sleep.

Breathwork

As we saw in Chapter 2, sleep isn't just about what we do in the evening – it's about what we do around the clock. This week, we're going to be taking a much more holistic approach to sleeping better – starting from the moment you wake up. We'll start each day with a simple "belly breathing" exercise.

1. Close your eyes and lie on your back with your hands placed on your belly.

2. Inhale through your nose for the count of five. Let your belly rise as it fills up. If you're just starting this technique, it might take a bit of practice to guide your breath into your stomach rather than just your chest.

3. Let the breath flow softly out for a count of eight, emptying your belly. Let go of any anxiety about the day ahead.

4. Feel your stomach rise and fall beneath your hands with each breath.

5. Do this for ten rounds.

You might also like to repeat one of your morning affirmations as you do this, to set yourself up for the day.

Evening Affirmation

These are simple things to do at the end of the day to switch off before bed. Better to practise these than fall down a rabbit hole on your phone!

1. I'm feeling peaceful and calm.

2. With every breath, I feel myself relax.

3. I am not defined by whatever happened today; I choose to let go and surrender.

4. I let go of every worry. My eyes, mind and body are tired, and I deserve a night of relaxing sleep.

5. I did my best today, my body is ready to rest. Tomorrow is a new day.

If my head is too busy to focus, I come back to my keywords: cool, calm, collected, confident and courageous. Try not to over-analyse your sleep patterns or get caught up in how much you're *not* sleeping. Remember, rest is still beneficial for your body – even if you're not asleep.

Nutrition

Having spent last week focusing on some basics of what to eat and what not to eat, this week we're going to look at *when* you eat to promote better sleep. If you're a coffee lover but are struggling to sleep, let's stick to one caffeine hit a day. Have one proper cup of coffee and enjoy it. No lattes, or Frappuccinos®, or gingerbread mega whappuccinos!

If you're more of a tea person, remember that black tea also contains caffeine. Tea and coffee also don't make up your daily water consumption. They're diuretics (meaning they cause more urine to pass out of the body), so can actually dehydrate you.

The amount of time it takes for our bodies to process caffeine varies from person to person. As a rule of thumb, let's say no caffeinated drinks after 3pm. If you feel like you can cut caffeine out completely, then go for it. Just be aware that you might get headaches and feel grumpy for a couple of days as your body goes through a withdrawal process. Whether you're cutting out or simply reducing your caffeine intake, drinking plenty of water is key.

It's a cliché, but try having a chamomile tea before bedtime. My grandmother got me into this habit and it's been part of my evening routine for decades. It calms the mind and body and has anti-inflammatory properties. Some research even suggests that chamomile has similar effects to benzodiazepine – a prescription drug that reduces anxiety and induces sleep.

Top five foods to avoid before bedtime

Raw vegetables

Despite being packed with antioxidants, vitamins and minerals, they don't help you sleep at night. Raw foods are more difficult to break down and you may experience flatulence or bloating, which prevents you from falling asleep.

Raw cruciferous vegetables such as broccoli, cabbage and Brussel sprouts are the worst offenders, so steer clear of them at least three hours before bedtime.

Chocolate

This has been my downfall on many occasions! Having treated myself to some dark chocolate after my evening meal, I've found myself wide awake into the early hours of the morning. Good-quality dark chocolate that's rich in cacao has many beneficial nutrients, but it also brings a hefty hit of caffeine. And, as the percentage of cacao increases, so too does the caffeine content. A 1.5 ounce serving of 80 per cent cacao chocolate provides around 40–75mg of caffeine. This is quite impressive when you consider that coffee contains between 100–300mg of caffeine per 8 ounces. Like caffeinated drinks, restrict your chocolate intake to before 3pm.

Dried fruit

Dried fruit is high in dietary fibre, but it's also packed with natural sugar: fructose. In small amounts, fructose is fine. However, if you're digging into a whole bag of dried apricots before bed, don't be surprised if your sleep is disturbed. Too much fibre can easily upset your digestive system, not to mention the fact that sugar raises your blood glucose levels, making it harder for you to get to sleep. Like cruciferous vegetables, dried apricots can also cause wind.

Cheese

Many people see cheese as comfort food. But it's one of the worst things you can eat before bedtime, as it can give you crazily vivid dreams. Strong or aged cheese, as well as preserved meats such as bacon, ham and pepperoni, contain naturally high levels of the amino acid tyramine. Tyramine causes the adrenal gland to release the fight-or-flight hormone, which increases alertness for several hours.

Crisps/salted nuts

Too much salt dehydrates the body and increases water retention, causing tiredness and fatigue. A study by the European Society of Endocrinology found that salty foods, such as crisps and salted nuts, were some of the worst foods to eat before bed as they contributed to disrupted – or "superficial" – sleep. Stay away from salty foods at least two to three hours before bed.

Top three foods for good sleep (also better skin!)

Raw honey

Honey stimulates melatonin and shuts off orexin – the neuropeptide that makes us feel sharp and alert. A mug of hot water, lemon and honey is a great evening drink for soothing the body and inducing sleep. My grandmother would always give us a cup of warm milk or chamomile tea and honey before bedtime as children and it's something I continued with my kids. Now that there are so many dairy alternatives on the market, I've switched from regular milk to nut milks.

Bananas

Although they contain fruit sugar, bananas bring other benefits. If you usually have a banana for breakfast, try switching things up and having it before bedtime this week. Bananas contain high levels of magnesium, which relaxes our muscles and calms the body. Try some sliced banana with a tablespoon of natural nut butter as a bedtime snack. My kids can always tell if I've had a sleepless night, as the banana skin will be left out on the kitchen worktop!

Almonds

Just like bananas, almonds are great for a good night's sleep as they contain high levels of melatonin – the hormone that helps regulate our sleep/wake cycle. A 1oz serving of whole almonds also contains 77mg of magnesium and 76mg of calcium. Both of these minerals may help promote muscle relaxation and sleep.

Supplements for stress relief and better sleep

Even with the best-laid plans and good habits throughout the day, we all suffer from poor sleep from time to time. As someone who has suffered from sleep problems periodically throughout my life, these supplements are the ones I've personally found to be particularly good at helping me get a good night's rest – without the "hangover" effect.

Magnolia bark: the extract of Magnolia bark *(Magnolia officianalis)* is native to China and has been used in traditional Eastern medicine for centuries. It works as what's known an "anxiolytic" – meaning it helps lower anxiety. Some research suggests that it may even suppress adrenalin and cortisol, and act as a sedative, thereby helping us relax and drift off to sleep.

Melatonin: as we know from Chapter 2, melatonin is the body's natural "sleep hormone". Certain lifestyle factors – including our age, weight, diet, sleep/wake cycle and exposure to (digital) light at night time – can inhibit the natural production of melatonin and compromise our sleep. We can take a man-made version in the form of supplements to help bolster these levels. It is, however, only available on prescription in the UK.

Asphalia for natural sleep: this plant-based supplement that I was recommended years ago from a naturopath has been one of those that has been a staple in my bedside drawer and when I travel. Being totally honest I don't fully understand how it benefits, it just does! It contains an antioxidant that's five times as powerful as vitamin C and possibly 500 times more potent than most synthetic antioxidants. It works by regulating our natural sleep cycle, helping us get a good night's rest without disturbance.

Vitamin N

This week, I want you to bring the outside in. We can do this in a variety of ways, depending on what's available to you. You may want to try introducing a house plant into your living space. Maybe you want to fill your whole bathroom with plants! If this isn't possible for you, then how about drawing it in pencil, biro, paints, chalks – or whatever you have access to? It might be a quick doodle or a two-hour art session. You can try having a plant in front of you, print a picture from the Internet, or simply use your imagination.

House plants have been proven to reduce stress and anxiety and boost our mood. The process of feeding, watering and nurturing plants is also cathartic. These are all things we need to do for ourselves if we want to thrive!

Physical Support: Cold Bathing/Showering

Now, it's time for your real wake-up call! As part of Week 2, we're going to start each day with a cold shower or bath. Check back with the guidance in Chapter 3 if you need tips. Then, just do it! Write down how you find the experience, comparing the beginning of the week to the end.

Physical Activity

This week, we're focusing on loosening up your joints and re-energizing your body. You'll need a place with sufficient space to perform these dynamic stretches. Unlike static stretches (which involve holding one position for several seconds), dynamic stretching uses active movement. They can also be performed as a warm-up before exercise.

Stretch 1

1. Stand with your feet shoulder-width apart, tailbone tucked under (make sure your bottom is not jutting out, creating a curve in your lower back) and hold your arms out to the side at shoulder height.

2. Make small circles with your arms. Do twenty in one direction and twenty in the other.

3. Repeat the process, this time making larger and larger circles as you go.

Stretch 2

1. Start as you did in stretch 1.

2. Root your feet down, keep your hips facing forward and your arms dangling loosely by your sides.

3. Twist your upper body from side to side, allowing your arms and hands to swing. Keep your hips square to create a stretch across the middle of your body.

4. Repeat twenty times, making your rotations bigger and more dynamic as you go. If you get dizzy, keep your head facing forward.

Stretch 3

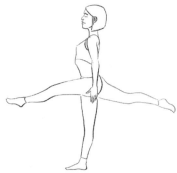

1. Hold onto something with one hand (make sure you have enough space around you!) and swing your opposite leg forward and back, as high as it will go without letting your pelvis tip forward or back or from one side to the other. Keep your core engaged to prevent your back from curving. Ten swings each leg.

Stretch 4

1. With your legs together, start performing small jumps. If this feels too much, just come onto your tiptoes and back down again. Do fifty repetitions.

Stretch 5

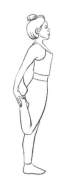

1. Stand with your feet hip-width apart, using one hand on a wall or surface to support you.

2. Bend the opposite leg, squeezing your knee to your chest.

3. Take the same leg to your bottom, moving your heel toward your bottom, pressing your foot or lower leg into your bottom to create a stretch. Hold each forward and backward movement for a moment to create a stretch.

4. Repeat five times on each side.

Stretch 6

1. Bend into a forward fold, placing your palms on the floor. Walk out your legs, with your knees bent.

Stretch 7

1. Step back into a downward dog.

2. Paddle out your legs.

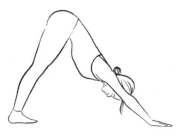 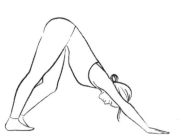

3. Bend your knees, then push up onto tiptoes, shining your tailbone to the sky.

4. Spread your fingertips out evenly, nod your head "yes", shake your head "no".

5. Find stillness for five breaths.

Stretch 8

1. Step your right leg forward into a low lunge.

2. Drop your left knee to the floor and bring your arms up above your head, placing your palms together.

3. Hold for three breaths.

4. Place your hands on either side of your right foot.

5. Raise your left knee off the ground, holding that leg firm.

6. Keeping your left hand on the floor, rotate your body and raise your right arm to the sky. Hold for three breaths.

7. Step back into downward dog.

8. Repeat on the other side.

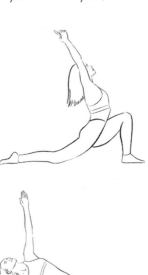

Stretch 9

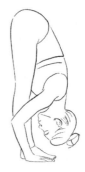

1. Return to downward dog.

2. Walk your hands back toward your feet so you're in a forward fold with your knees bent.

3. Slowly stand up, rolling up – vertebra by vertebra – until you're upright.

4. Place your hands in prayer and take three to five full breaths.

Skincare

Along with setting your body up for better sleep, Week 2 of the plan focuses on your evening skincare routine.

Essentials:

- Cleanse every evening but NO FACE WIPES!

- Ensure you remove your eye make-up thoroughly – but don't rub your eyes/lashes too harshly

- Ideally ditch micellar water, and only use it if other cleansers aren't available

- You only need to double cleanse if you're wearing make-up

- No eye creams at night, unless they are a retinoid product in a serum or light texture

Your evening skincare routine

I prefer to use a cleansing cloth with a splash of cold water or one press with a cold compress.

1. Cleanse

2. Face massage routine

3. Cleanse again (to remove any leftover oil)

4. Serum 1: a retinoid, peptide, stem cell, or something targeting a skin concern, such as a pigmentation or acne serum. You might find the skin comes up slightly pink with certain actives after you've done your facial massage.

5. No heavy night creams. Use either a drop of oil, a second hydrating serum or a hydrating tonic.

Optional

One to three nights a week, you can use an acid-based tonic after cleansing. Not all skins need them and some serums will contain acids. Avoid doubling up on acids.

Try a mask that's hydrating, calming and soothing.

Evening face massage

Use slow, deep movements that not only work on the physical tissues of your face, but also help to calm your mind. Avoid fast flicking motions, as they can stimulate the nervous system and prevent you from getting a good night's rest. Repeat every move five to ten times

Apply oil to your face and neck. You can do the neck stretches that we covered in Week 1 to ease out any tension from the day.

1. Using the palms of your hands, glide up the cheeks from your jaw to your cheekbone. Hold at the cheekbone then glide up to your temples. Repeat five times.

2. Start with your palms over your mouth and push upward and outward.

3. On one side of your face, use the opposite thumb to push out along your jawline. Then, use your knuckles on your other hand to glide outward from chin to ear. Alternate between pushing with your thumb and your knuckle.

4. Push upward from your jaw to your temples with the pads of your palms. Repeat four to five times on each side of your face.

5. Scissor your fingers as you glide around the sides of your mouth.

6. Glide over your cheekbones toward your ears five times.

7. Use your knuckles to create a "C" shape under your cheekbones, working from your nose to your ears and back again. Do both sides of your face at the same time.

8. Use one or two fingers to push your nasolabial line upward working toward your brows. Press up beneath your brow as you glide out toward your temples. Repeat five times.

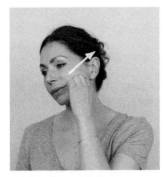

3b.

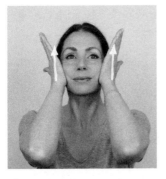

1.

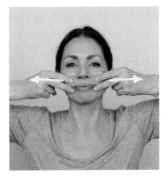

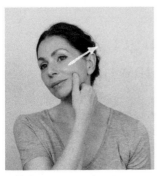

5.

3a.

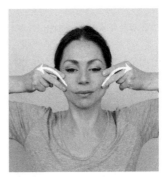

6.

9. Push up and hold beneath your brow for a count of five. Repeat on the other side.

10. Smooth up your brows using alternate hands.

11. Using firm pressure, glide your fingers up over your forehead, pressing into the hairline.

12. Slowly criss-cross your fingers over your forehead, focusing on the middle, where your "third eye" is.

13. Using a lighter pressure, criss-cross over your crow's feet, moving in an upward direction.

14. Scissor either side of your ears.

15. Glide out and down over your face and neck in a smoothing action.

16. Finish with light pumping motions above your clavicle.

···• This Week's Target Area: •··· Cheeks and Jawline

There are a lot of muscles to consider in this part of the face:

Chin: mentalis, depressor labii inferioris, depressor anguli oris

Cheeks: risorius, levator anguli oris, levator labii superioris, masseter, buccinator, zygomaticus

Mouth: orbicularis oris

Neck: platysma

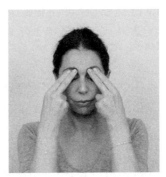

9.

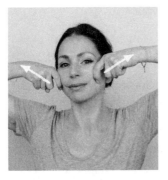

7.

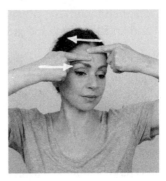

12.

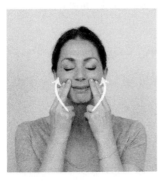

8.

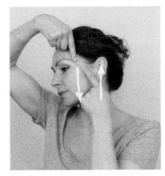

13.

Many of us experience loss of firmness around the jawline. Yet, facial massage is an effective way of softening and lifting these lines and restoring your skin's glow.

Key moves to refine your jawline – with oil

1. Knuckle gliding: use your fore and middle finger knuckles to glide outward from your chin to your ear.

2. Thumb pushes: support your chin with one hand and push out along the jaw, using the knuckle of the other hand.

3. Pinch flick: support the skin on your chin and neck with one hand. With the other hand, pinch flick with your thumb and knuckle along the jawline.

4. Flicking: support your skin with one hand. With the other hand, use two fingers to flick upward along your jaw.

5. Still hold: place one hand on your neck and the other above your jawline. Use the pads of your hands to lift and hold.

Key moves for your cheek area – with oil

Do the following exercises on one side of your face, then on the other side.

1. Cheek push-ups: glide upward and hold, using the pads of your hands.

2. Knuckle glide-ups: make a fist. Glide upward from your jawline to your cheekbone and hold. Rock back and forth under your cheekbones.

3. Flicking: support your skin with one hand. With the other hand, use two fingers to create firm, fast flicking motions across your entire cheek area.

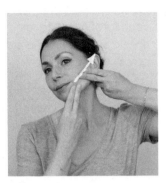

3.

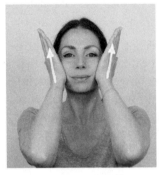

1.

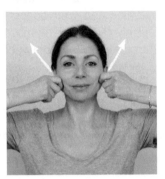

4.

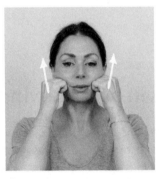

2.

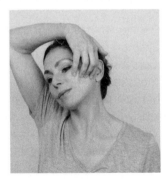

5.

4. Double hand flicks: use your thumbs and the knuckles of your forefingers to pinch, twist, lift and flick across your cheek. Start near the side of your mouth and move out across the cheek.

5. Take one hand over your head, so your fingers are lifting the skin of your cheek. Lift under and upward. Then finger walk along your cheek.

6. Sausage roll: place your hands in front of you, as if you're holding a burger (thumbs at the bottom, fingers together at the top, leaving space for the burger in the middle). Place this shape on one cheek, with your thumbs on your jawline and your fingers on your cheekbone. Slowly and firmly glide your thumbs up to meet your fingers, creating a sausage of skin between the two. Hold.

7. Full hand push-ups to the side of your face.

8. Full knuckle push-ups to the side of your face.

9. Quick, small finger pinching to whole area.

Lymphatics – Letting Go or "Detoxing"

We've already talked about the importance of lymphatic drainage in Chapter 7. Lymphatic drainage is a form of gentle massage that encourages the movement of lymph fluids around the body. These methods can be incredibly beneficial for skin health – even for those with a condition like acne or rosacea. Other forms of massage are generally too stimulating for these skin types.

Whether or not you have a skin condition, lymphatic drainage can be immensely calming and help reduce puffiness.

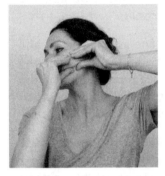

6.

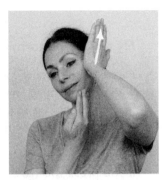

7b.

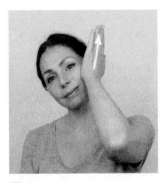

7a.

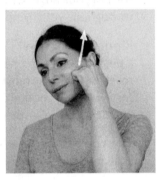

8a.

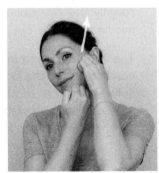

8b.

My tips for performing lymphatic drainage:

- Please note, many people online advise using oil when performing lymphatic drainage, but they're misinformed! The extra "slip" can mean we miss the all-important lymph and limit results.

- The lymphatic vessels are as fine as silk strands, and if you press too hard, you'll flatten them. Imagine the light pressure of a twenty-pence piece resting on the pads of your fingers, then try to recreate this sensation throughout your lymph drainage practice.

- Rhythm is king here! The lymphatic system doesn't have a pump (such as the heart) to move lymph around, so it relies on muscular movement and a very slight peristalsis (or wave-like) motion. Think about how dancers count "one, two, three" – then go even slower.

- The point is to move the skin over tissue, applying a little pressure before releasing.

- Direction – if you were to lay on your back and pour water on your face, the direction in which it falls is roughly the direction of lymphatic drainage: from the middle of the face, out to your ears and down your neck.

- The lymphatic system is a little like a traffic jam. We need to move the traffic at the front of the queue before the rest of the cars can continue on their journey. For this reason, we always start at the neck, then work up to the face, then back down again.

Lymphatic massage movements – pump in each place eight times

1. Starting on the sides of your neck, keep your hands flat as you pump downward from your ears. Keep your little fingers close to your ears.

2. Pump two fingers just above your clavicle.

3. Repeat steps 1 and 2 three times.

4. Place your finger pads on your chin and pump downward. Repeat this move in three more positions, working along your jaw toward your ears.

5. Place your fingertips just in front of your ears and pump downward.

6. Do the same in the middle of your cheeks.

7. Repeat under your eyes.

8. On your temples.

9. On your forehead.

10. Glide your flat hands outward across your forehead, moving down over your entire face. Repeat steps 1 and 2 on your neck.

You can repeat the above three times and focus on any areas of concern.

✦ Gadget Highlight: Cupping ✦

We talked about cupping in Chapter 7. Many people assume it's complicated, but really, once you get to grips with it, the method is relatively simple. Cupping brings fresh blood to the surface, can encourage drainage and reduce puffiness. Proceed with caution if you're prone to flushing as cupping very stimulating, so may increase redness. Otherwise, it's likely to leave you with a lovely rosy glow.

The key is to place the cup on your skin and squeeze only when you have full contact. You'll be able to tell because the cup will suck up a tiny bit of skin. Once this happens, glide the cup across your skin, then release and lift it off. Place the cup on your next target area – and repeat.

When cupping, we generally follow the same direction as we do when performing lymphatic drainage.

1. Start on your neck and glide outward from your chin to your jaw, and back down the sides of your neck.

2. Glide out across your jawline to your ear.

3. Glide from the sides of your mouth to your ears.

4. Under your cheekbones.

5. Gently under your eyes.

6. Out across one side of your forehead, then down the sides of your face and neck.

7. Repeat the above steps on the other side of your face.

8. Finish by gliding down the sides of your neck to your clavicles.

Colour Wheel Meditation for Better Sleep

This is one of my favourite techniques to use when I'm struggling to switch off. The combination of breathwork and visualisation is particularly useful if you find your mind racing at night.

I've called this a colour wheel meditation but it's also referred to as chakra meditation. It involves focusing on seven specific areas of the body while visualizing colours and wheel-like shapes. If you're into chakras and healing, each chakra has its own colour. Red and orange start at the tailbone; yellow, green, blue, indigo and violet follow as you move up toward the crown of your head.

As you focus on each area of the body during this exercise, imagine breathing in the colour we're focusing on.

1. Find a comfortable position, lying down or seated, and close your eyes.

2. Focus on your tailbone for the next five to ten breaths as you imagine a circle of warm red energy swirling around you.

3. Move your focus to your lower abdomen. Picture the colour orange circling around as you breathe for five to ten breaths.

4. Focus on the area just beneath your rib cage, otherwise known as the solar plexus. Imagine the colour yellow spinning for five to ten breaths.

5. Move your attention to the centre of your chest. Focus on a green circle of energy.

6. Focus now on the neck and the colour blue.

7. Move up to the area in the middle of your forehead known as the third eye. This time, the colour is indigo.

8. Finally, move up to the crown of your head. Imagine violet light.

Journalling

Now that you've been journalling for a fortnight, let's reflect on how it's affecting you and continue jotting things down. Here are some things you might like to cover.

- **How are you feeling after this week?**
- **How did you feel when you woke up this morning?**
- **How many hours of sleep did you get?**
- **What time did you go to bed?**
- **What wind-down routine did you do today?**
- **How did the stretches make you feel?**
- **Were they difficult or challenging?**
- **How did you feel before and after your cold bath?**

Congratulations on completing Week 2!

Some space for your thoughts

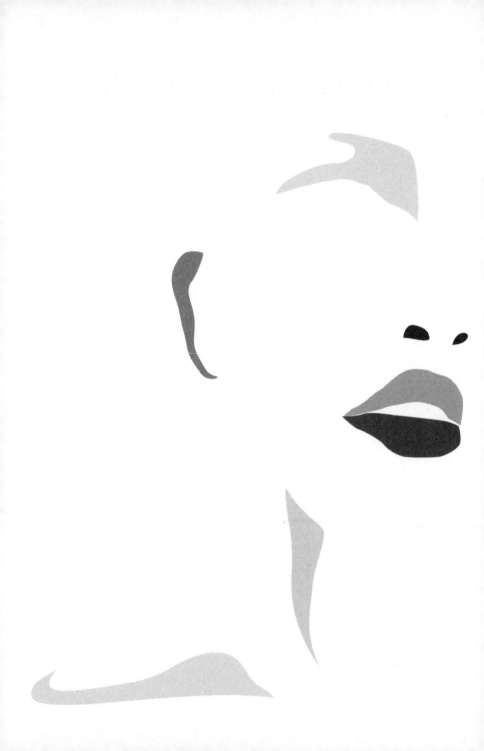

11

The Glow Plan: Week 3

Letting Go

Focus area: eyes, facial acupressure, gua sha

Letting go can be a fundamental part of finding more emotional stability, calm, happiness and acceptance; of being more comfortable in our own skin. It's actually an immensely difficult thing to do.

By letting go, I mean taking the time to consider ideas that we hold about ourselves and the world around us, then thinking about whether we'd benefit from looking at these very same perceptions through a different lens. When we let go of something that no longer serves us, it allows space for something new. It often involves things that have become so hardwired within our minds that we don't even realize they're holding us back.

The ageing process can be emotionally challenging at the best of times. It's hard to let go of our twenty-something looks and accept a new type of beauty that we encounter with each decade.

Things to let go of this week:

- Social stereotypes about what we should or shouldn't look like

- Pressure to be flawless and perfect

- Not being allowed to embrace your natural hair

- Feeling less confident because your face and body has changed

- Habits that harm your skin and wellbeing

- Feeling guilty

So, this week we're going to build on the morning and evening routines we established in weeks 1 and 2, with a bit more focus on letting go. Journalling is particularly important this week.

Gratitude

This week I'm thankful for my skin. It protects me from external things and keeps my organs safe.

I'm thankful I can read and learn more about my body and the world around me.
I find joy in the small things in life.
I am so grateful for all the love in my life.
Today, I am grateful for (list three things) …
Three of my most precious possessions are …

Happiness

List three things that have made you smile.

Affirmations

I let go of comparison.
I let go of fear, judgement, others' opinions, indecision, shame.
I let go of the need to control situations.
I let go of hurt from the past.
I'm open to new possibilities and opportunities.

Breathwork

Open breath is a powerful tool that you can turn to whenever you need to release tension and stress. It's particularly useful for those moments when you're feeling stuck, anxious or overwhelmed, and need to let go. Focus on opening your mouth on the exhale.

1. Find a comfortable seat or lie down. Allow your body to relax.

2. Take a deep inhale through your nose to a count of six until you reach about 70 per cent lung capacity.

3. As you inhale, imagine you're inhaling a positive, uplifting quality, such as ease, peace, calm or a bright, happy colour.

4. Hold the breath for one to two counts at the top.

5. Now exhale with your mouth open, imagining that you're releasing whatever no longer serves you; this might be physical tension, stress, pain, sadness, worry, a memory, a thought, or whatever you would like to release.

6. You can push the breath out through your lips or just let it out through your throat.

7. Go right to the bottom of the exhalation.

8. Repeat this cycle for three to five minutes.

Notice how your mind and body feel afterwards. Can you sense some kind of release, lightness or newfound energy?

———————————

Nutrition

This week, I want you to focus on the balance of your diet. Are you eating a lot of bread, cereal, pasta and sugary snacks each day? Do you really need that second latte? Can you add some more foods from the "good for gut health" list – and cut down/remove some others? It's worth considering some simple switch-ups to regain balance and support your gut. Remember, a healthy gut is better able to absorb nutrients from the rest of the diet – so even small changes can make a difference.

Foods for good gut health

live yoghurt	leeks
kefir	onions
sauerkraut	raspberries
kimchi	bananas
kombucha	pears
tempeh	broccoli
miso	lentils
Jerusalem artichokes	chickpeas
asparagus	beans (kidney, pinto and white)
wholegrains	green tea

Foods to reduce or avoid

alcohol	artificial sweeteners
sugar	refined food (white carbohydrates)
fried food	processed food and meat

Food switch-ups

In Chapter 5, we looked at the link between gut health, inflammation and cellular ageing. Now, we're going to put this into practice with some simple food switch-ups that support your gut.

Remember that your microbiome is unique, so what works for me might not be best for you. Fermented foods can irritate a sensitive gut; kefir (a fermented yoghurt drink) is great – unless you're lactose intolerant. Miso and tempeh are fermented soy – some people have a sensitivity to soy. You'll need to experiment a little to find out what works for you. The most effective way to find out what's going on in your gut is to have a stool test with a registered nutritionist.

Dairy

Dairy isn't "bad" for you (unless you're allergic or intolerant to lactose). However, many of us tend to overdo it, drinking lattes and eating cheese, yoghurt and milk in excess. I love a good-quality organic milk – and in my view, a proper English cuppa wouldn't be the same without it – but there are also great lactose-free milk options. It's worth considering some of the dairy alternatives.

Hemp milk: highest in protein and healthy omega fats, low in carbohydrates – it's great for your skin.

Oat milk: higher in carbohydrates, it contains a good amount of soluble fibre, which helps stabilize blood sugar levels and cholesterol while keeping you feeling fuller for longer.

Almond milk: lower in protein carbohydrates than some other milks, it contains antioxidant vitamin E – and is often fortified with nutrients such as calcium, as well as vitamins A and D.

Coconut milk: contains even less protein than almond milk, but is often fortified with other nutrients. It's higher in fat than some milks and contains medium-chain triglycerides (MCTs), which have been linked to improved heart health.

Soy milk: an excellent source of protein, soy milk closely resembles the nutritional make-up of cow's milk and has been linked to improved cholesterol and blood pressure levels. Try and pick organic soy milk made from non-genetically modified soy beans without the use of conventional pesticides and herbicides.

Gluten

Gluten has quite clearly been linked to a number of digestive disorders. It's commonly found in bread, pasta, pizza, cereal – and even many household condiments, such as soy sauce and some salad dressings. People with Coeliac disease suffer from an immune reaction that's triggered by eating gluten. They develop inflammation in their intestinal tracts and other parts of the body.

Coeliac disease is still relatively uncommon (it affects around 1 per cent of the UK population). My grandmother was coeliac, so gluten free is something my family have been familiar with well before it became fashionable! Some people are "gluten sensitive" – in my case my sensitivity is with yeast and raising agents. If you are experience cramping, pain, bloating, constipation and/or diarrhoea, you may want to try cutting out anything containing gluten to see how you feel and also chat with a nutritionist; there are tests which can be done to rule out allergies and also establish sensitivities.

Allergy v intolerance: what's the difference?

When considering your food switch-ups this week, it's important to keep the difference between food intolerances and allergies in mind. An allergy triggers an immune system response that manifests as symptoms that can be severe, or even life-threatening.

An intolerance, on the other hand, will cause more minor symptoms: bloating, diarrhoea, constipation and cramping, along with brain fog, lethargy and joint aches. Most people can eat a little of a food they're intolerant to but find that larger quantities will set off their symptoms. Intolerances are often caused by a lack of an enzyme required to digest a certain food type (as with lactose) or by a sensitivity to certain additives (such as the sulphates in canned goods, dried fruit and vinegar). Stress and anxiety can also play a role in triggering intolerances and digestive flare-ups. The best way to find out if you're allergic or intolerant to certain foods is to take a professional sensitivity test.

Vitamin N: Cloudscaping

If like me, you grew up in the UK, you'll be familiar with cloudy days! Cloudscaping is something I did as a child – just lying on my back and gazing up at the sky, imagining what shapes and pictures I could see in the clouds. I've cloudscaped on teenage dates, on long car journeys with my children and while sunbathing as an adult. It's accessible to everyone – and you're never too young or too old to start!

I find cloudscaping immensely calming – especially if your mind is in overdrive and you want to switch off. It's a way of connecting with nature, which brings myriad health benefits.

If you'd like more tips, take a look at The Cloud Appreciation Society website. They also have their own Instagram handle: @cloudappsoc

---

Physical Support

Continue body brushing and cold bathing, as you did in weeks 1 and 2. This week, we'll add hand reflexology moves into your routine, three times a week – or more. Make them a habit that you do in the shower, while sitting on the bus or walking in the park. It only takes two minutes to massage your hands – so stop scrolling on your phone and take a moment to care for yourself!

It might seem odd to focus on your hands. But think how much they do for you on a daily basis. Hand reflexology is a simple way of showing them some love by easing out all the tension they hold. Like our face, our hands are exposed to the elements, so are vulnerable to the signs of ageing – even more of a reason to give them some TLC! Also, hand reflexology has a physical impact on your muscles and is scientifically proven to help ease stress and boost your mood. You can do this routine with a cream or oil.

1. With your hands clasped together, stretch your arms away from you so all your fingers stretch backward. This is also nice to do above your head, stretching your arms up to the ceiling.

2. Bend each of your fingers back, one at a time.

3. Hold all your fingers together and gently pull them back toward your body to feel a gentle stretch.

4. Use your thumb to push up in a caterpillar massage motion from the bottom of your palm to the base of each finger and thumb.

5. Wring and twist down each of your fingers and thumb from the knuckle to the tips using the opposite hand.

6. Press your thumb right into the middle of your other palm (this point is called the plexus).

Hand reflexology points for overall health

Kidney/adrenals: pads of your thumbs

Head and neck: length and tips of your thumbs

Lymphatic: back of your hand and in the spaces between tendons

Stomach: the webbed area between your thumb and forefinger

Small intestine and large: outer and lower pads

Liver spleen: the padded area on the side of your hand

Physical Activity

You can continue with the stretches we covered in weeks 1 and 2. This week, we're going to add to those by getting your heart rate pumping with some jumping, skipping and rebounding.

As you know from Chapter 3, there are endless benefits to increasing your movement and boosting your cardiovascular health. Whether you skip, jump or rebound, you can easily tailor the intensity to suit your body (yes, even if you have dodgy knees/pelvic floor!). Just think of your exercise as playtime, and embrace it with joy, as you would have done as a child. Don't worry about what you look like – it's time to let your inhibitions go.

The benefits are an increased heart rate, coordination, concentration and improved mental health. It also supports the lymphatic system, general physical fitness and puts a smile on your face!

Do one of the below for 100 repetitions each morning. If you want to – and feel able – do more than 100.

Level 1 – tiptoe jumps: with your feet hip-width apart, make a jumping motion but keep your toes on the floor. Come up onto the balls of your feet and back down again, bending your knees each time.

Level 2 – small jumps: support your boobs by holding onto them if you need to!

Level 3 – rebounding: jumps can be fast or slow. If you're a beginner, you might start with low jumps then build toward bigger movements as you gain confidence and balance.

Level 4 – skipping: you'll be amazed by how challenging skipping is, compared to jumping. If you don't have a skipping rope, start by performing the action with your legs and arms. The movement of your arms is important as it dramatically increases your heart rate.

Deep Dive: Facial Tissue

The face isn't just made up of skin, bone and muscle; it's a lot more complex than that. The soft tissues of the face are arranged in a series of layers:

1. The skin – a complex organ which in itself consists of multiple layers

2. Subcutaneous fat

3. Superficial fascia, including platysma and the SMAS layer

4. Deep fascia

5. Deep muscle

6. Deep fat

7. Bone

Looking after our face and ageing well requires us to act on much more than the surface layer.

This Week's Target Area: Eyes

The eye contour is often where we first notice the signs of ageing, and it's a difficult area to treat.

Let's talk about dark circles

Dark circles are often hereditary and are caused by a slight change in the colour of the pigment in the skin beneath our eyes. As the skin here is thinner, when the blood vessels dilate (which happens when we're tired), they become more visible, forming dark, blueish circles.

What causes dark circles?

- dehydration
- lack of sleep
- allergies to foods such as gluten or dairy
- too much caffeine
- medication
- nutritional deficiencies

Nutritional deficiencies

When we're anaemic, our blood cells are unable to carry enough oxygen to the body's tissues – including those under the eyes. This can result in dark eye circles. Other vitamin deficiencies, including vitamin B12, E, K and D, have also been associated with dark circles.

Skincare: Eye Products

If you're in search of the Holy Grail here, I'm sorry to disappoint you, but I consider most eye products to be distinctly underwhelming! Almost all skincare brands have at least one eye product and recommend you apply it morning and night. Some of this is just marketing spin.

Time and time again, my clients come into the clinic concerned about puffy eyes. After a little investigation, it more often than not turns out that they've started using an eye product at night. When they switch products and ditch the heavy creams, they almost always see a dramatic reduction in puffiness.

The only eye products I use in the evening are retinoid-based formulas with a light, gel-like texture. If your eyes are still puffy in the morning, then get rid of your evening eye product and stick to using one in the morning. If you're currently using an eye product, I would like you to use it in the morning only for the rest of this plan.

Face Massage

The primary muscle associated with the eye area is the orbicularis oculi. It's a circular muscle that surrounds the eye and is connected to the frontalis and corrugator supercilii muscles (on the forehead and sides of the nose).

There are three parts to the orbicularis oculi, and one of its main functions is to allow us to blink, squint and wink. The movement of the muscles within our cheeks and forehead also supports other expressions around the eye area, such as raising our brows and smiling.

While on most of the body the skin is 2–3mm thick, under the eyes it's as thin as 0.5mm. And, unlike the rest of the skin on your face, the areas surrounding your eyes have no oil glands, so tend to become dry more easily.

People on social media have called me out several times because I have "wrinkly eyes". I'm totally fine with this as it's part of my genetics. Look at my family and you'll see the same thing. My advice would be to take ownership of your genes without judgement. I'm Caucasian and have a tendency toward dry skin and smiley eyes. It's all part of being me!

Of course, I can treat my eye area with products and massage. But I also need to be realistic about my goals if I still want to look natural as I age. Be warned: there's a growing number of people on social media (who are either too young to have developed crow's feet or are just genetically blessed in that area) making wild claims about the results massage will achieve. I prefer to be honest and say that whatever you do, you still need to take your genetics and lifestyle into account when thinking about what's realistic.

From my decades of hands-on experience, I believe the following is possible:

- a brighter eye area

- a wider, open-eyed look

- a reduction in puffiness

- a softer, more relaxed look to the eyes

- a softening of expression lines

- a more vibrant, youthful appearance

Massage moves for the eye area

You can be relatively firm here – just keep your movements short and controlled. Seeing the skin wrinkle a little as you perform these moves is absolutely fine. Dragging the skin in any way is not!

Without oil

1. **Eyelid push-ups:** place your finger pads onto your eyelids to create a slight resistance. With your eyes closed, look up and down five times.

2. **Owl eyes:** use your hands to make a "C" shape above and below your eyes, with your fingers above your brows and your thumbs just above your cheekbones. Press into the skin to create resistance as you squint and control the release slowly.

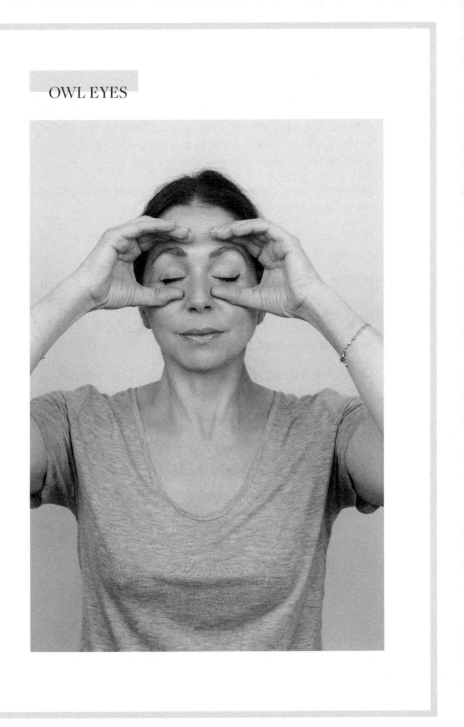

With oil – tap and glide to apply it

1. Using two fingers, trace around the eye area. Circle from the outer to the inner corner, then push up beneath the brows as you continue round. I use two fingers when pushing up and one finger when gliding under my eye.

2. Follow the same circle, but reverse the motion, moving from the inner corner out.

3. Using your middle fingers, rub firmly on the inner eye on the side of your nose to release tension.

4. Place the flat of one finger under your brow and push upward. Use the forefinger of the other hand to rub back and forth above the brow.

5. Pinch and lift outward across the brow.

6. Crow's feet: support your skin with one hand. Use the fingers of your opposite hand to glide upward over this area.

7. Finger walk: criss-cross over your crow's feet in an upward motion.

8. Repeat steps 1 to 7.

9. Drum your fingers over your entire face. Then use your hands to glide outward and downward in a smoothing motion.

MASSAGE MOVES: EYE AREA – WITH OIL

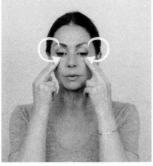

1.

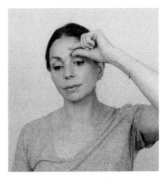

5.

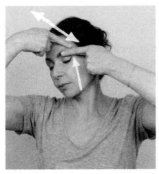

4.

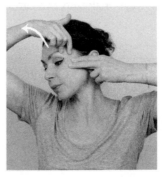

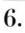

6.

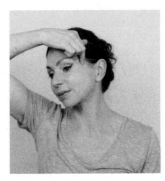

7.

What causes puffy eyes?

- too much coffee
- an underlying irritation to a skincare or make-up ingredient
- undiagnosed blepharitis
- a generally poor diet
- medication/drugs
- eye make-up can often cause irritation

A NOTE ON EYE MAKE-UP

I have to be immensely careful with eye make-up. I can be fine throughout the day, but by the following morning my skin may feel delicate and my eyes look swollen. Choosing mineral or properly natural/organic eye make-up has been a game-changer.

I recommend the following brands: ILIA, bareMinerals, RMS Beauty, Absolution, Kosas, Lily Lolo, Ere Perez, Vapour Beauty.

My tips to reduce puffy eyes:

- A cold compress – or even better, an ice compress: wrap an ice cube in tissue (don't put the naked cube on your skin) and glide it around your eyes. Gently pat and repeat.

- Cold spoons from the fridge – not freezer: glide them over your eyelids.

- Lymphatic pumps: place two or three fingers directly under your eyes using barely any pressure at all. Gently pump using a downward motion, then release the skin. Move your fingers out half a centimetre (toward your ears) and repeat. Move your fingers down, closer to your cheekbone and repeat.

- Repeat the same move with one finger right by the sides of your nose, close to your eye. Continue the delicate pumping action down the sides of your nose.

- Place your finger pads close to the outer edge of your eyes and pump. Finish with glides down the side of your face toward your ears.

Facial Acupressure

Acupressure follows the same principles as acupuncture, except it uses fingers rather than needles. It's deeply calming, and I love including it in my night-time skincare routine. The technique involves stimulating the internal organs via chi channels (meridians).

To perform facial acupressure, use your thumb or a finger to press firmly into each point. You can rotate or pump on each point, or just hold for five to ten seconds while breathing deeply and slowly. Don't worry about finding the exact point: you'll be stimulating local nerves and tissues even if you're not on the perfect spot.

Benefits

Improves circulation, releases tension within muscles and frees the flow of energy and blood. As most of these meridians begin and end on the face, you're also stimulating other areas of the body to soothe inflammation and support detoxification. By promoting blood flow at the skin surface, facial acupressure encourages all-important nutrients to reach our skin cells. This helps stimulate collagen production, increasing the elasticity of our skin and smoothing wrinkles.

Acupressure points

This can be done without oil at any time of the day. I like to use this method before and/or after my evening massage routine (see diagram and method).

If you're unsure of the exact acupressure points, spread your fingers as if holding a grapefruit in both hands and place them over your face. Keep all your fingers firm and press them over your face and scalp. Hold for a count of five. Repeat as you move around the face. This a fantastic way to relax before bed.

✧ Gadget Highlight: Gua Sha ✧

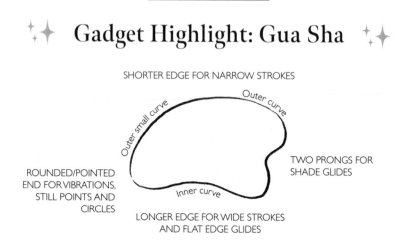

SHORTER EDGE FOR NARROW STROKES

Outer small curve

Outer curve

ROUNDED/POINTED END FOR VIBRATIONS, STILL POINTS AND CIRCLES

Inner curve

TWO PRONGS FOR SHADE GLIDES

LONGER EDGE FOR WIDE STROKES AND FLAT EDGE GLIDES

My tips for using a gua sha:

- Apply oil to your skin – too much, and there won't be enough friction; too little, and you risk dragging your skin.

- Always start with some neck drainage.

- Glide outward and downward.

- The speed, angle and duration change the results.

- Much of the method will be dictated by the bone structure of your face, which can act as a nice guide.

- Use the edge of the gua sha as it gives more focus and moves less tissue, which is good for lifting.

- Continue into your hairline with each movement.

- At the end of each glide (usually at the point of muscle attachment), wiggle the tool, as this can aid drainage.

Gua sha moves

Wide stroke: use the longer edge at an angle and medium pressure.

Flat edge glide: a wide stroke but at a closer angle to the skin.

Narrow stroke: use the shorter edge to focus on smaller areas.

Vibration: move the rounded end in a back and forth motion.

Still points: press the rounded end into a fixed point and hold for five to ten seconds.

Circles: lightly move the rounded end in circular motions.

Shape glide: glide the two prongs along the bone.

Zigzag: glide across your cheeks, chin and forehead.

Remember to work upward from your neck to your jaw, lower cheeks, upper cheeks, eyes and forehead. Then drain back down.

···• Your gua sha routine •···

Neck and head

1. Wide stroke up and down your neck, including the back.

2. Shape glide using a vibration method around the base of the occipital (the dip at the back of your head).

3. Shape glide in rows, working from your hairline to the back of your head.

4. Vibration in front of your ears and under your cheekbones. Then glide around your ears and down your neck.

Cheeks

1. Glide the flat edge in three to four rows across your jawline, moving from your chin to your ear, the side of your mouth to your ear, underneath your cheekbones and under your eye. Circle on your temples into your hairline.

2. Shape glide following the same path, supporting your skin with your free hand.

3. Using the curved edge, make small glides along the nasolabial line, supporting the skin on your lips with your free hand.

NECK AND HEAD

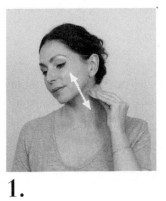

1.

CHEEKS

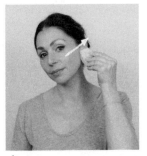

1a.

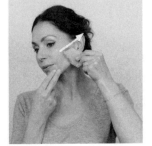

1b.

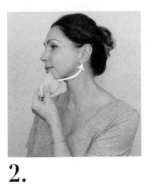

2.

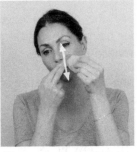

3.

4. Look up and do wide strokes up and down your neck.

5. Repeat all these moves on the other side.

Eyes

1. Using the outer curved edge, glide out and up under your eyes, from the sides of your nose to your temples.

2. Raise one brow and support it with your free hand. Use the tool to glide underneath the brow.

3. Vibrate at your temples.

4. Lift your brow with one flat finger: vibrate just above the brow, making horizontal rows that move from your brow to your hairline until you've covered your entire forehead.

Mouth

1. Using the small curved edge, glide outward from the midline of your lips. Work above your mouth, then below. Repeat on the other side. Support your skin with your free hand.

2. Using the curved tip, circle across your upper lip.

3. Vibrate on your chin and under the lip area.

Forehead

1. Using the pronged edge, glide up from your brows to your hairline in vertical rows. Repeat, covering the entire forehead three times.

2. Using the curved edge, vibrate in circular rows from your brow to your hairline.

EYES

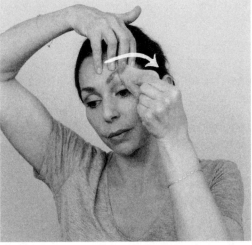

2.

FOREHEAD

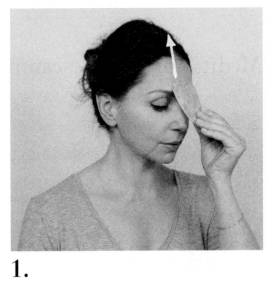

1.

3. Use the inner curve flat edge to glide up over your entire forehead.

4. Change direction to glide outward from midline out on both sides.

Décolleté

1. Using the large outer curve, glide and drain down the middle of your chest.

2. Use the same edge to glide out in three rows from the middle of your chest to your armpits.

A NOTE ON
JADE ROLLERS

I find gua shas more effective than jade rollers. However, if a roller is your preference, you can repeat all of the above moves to perform lymphatic drainage, always remembering to start at your neck and work upward.

Meditation – body scanning

1. Find somewhere comfortable to sit or lie down.

2. Take a few deep breaths, in and out of your nose.

3. As you exhale, let go of anything that's on your mind.

4. Let go of any tension in the body; zone out of the noises around you; drop your shoulders, soften your jaw.

5. Take a deep inhale.

6. As you exhale, allow your eyes to close.

7. Feel the weight of your body sink into whatever you're lying or sitting on. Let your mind relax and do its own thing; just allow thoughts to come and go.

8. Pay attention to your body. Does it feel light or heavy? Restless or still? Do you feel irritated or at ease?

9. Starting from the crown of your head, slowly scan down your body, turning your attention to your head, neck, arms, hands, chest, stomach, buttocks, thighs, knees, calves and ankles, until you get to your feet and toes. Just notice what feels tense and what feels at ease.

10. Keep your focus on your body, letting your mind do whatever it wants to do. As you scan, pay attention to the rise and fall of your chest and the sensation of your breath.

11. If you experience a thought or a feeling, just label it. Don't attempt to push it away. Acknowledge it.

12. Give your mind lots of space and freedom to do what it wants. Just try and remain focused on the breath as you continue the body scan.

13. Notice anything that you're holding onto. Any stories that you're telling yourself. Let the stories go.

14. Work your way down the body several times, at your own pace, noticing everything you experience.

15. Come back to the sensation of your breath. Observe anything that's shifted in your mind and body.

16. Take a deep inhale. Let the breath out through your mouth for a count of four and gently open your eyes.

Journalling

- One positive attribute about myself is ...

- Today, I choose to let go of three things that I can't control, including ...

- Rather than doubting myself, I trust that no matter what happens I will ...

- When I am finally able to let go of <fill in>, I will feel ...

- Something that didn't work out in the past was <fill in>, but I am grateful it didn't because ...

- I choose to create more space in my life for ...

- When I think about letting go of <insert negative habit>, I feel ...

- Make a note of something from this week you are proud of.

Congratulations on completing Week 3! This is often the most challenging, so well done! Only seven more days to go!

Some space for your thoughts

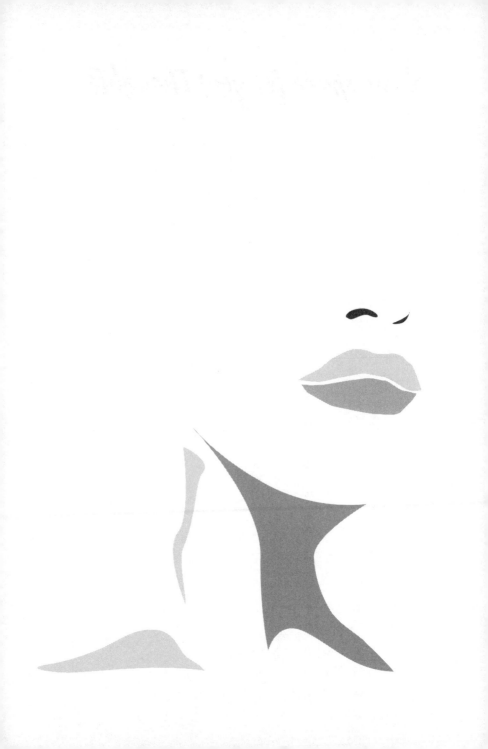

12

The Glow Plan: Week 4

Self-love

Focus area: mouth/lips/nasolabial lines

Self-love can feel like an elusive goal. It takes time – and needs dedication and commitment if we're to achieve it. Yet, I believe that it's an integral part of ageing well. How can we possibly *look* beautiful if we don't *feel* beautiful? Being highly self-critical for much of the time leads to emotional stress and a loss of self-confidence. It's all too easy to get trapped in a vicious cycle.

Self-love is something I've struggled with for a long time. Externally, I may come across as confident and in control of my life, but on the inside, that isn't always the case. I have a past, with many failings; plus, working in the beauty industry has sometimes made me feel under even more pressure to look a certain way or be a font of eternal youth. In the past, I've used filters on social media posts to hide my embarrassment about how old I felt my face looked or because I wasn't happy with my body shape. It's taken many years of learning, practising yoga and emotional growth to reach a place where I feel more content and am gentler to myself.

As humans, we are all imperfect. So, why is it that we strive for perfection? It's time to reframe our mindset, embrace our imperfections and find a calmer, kinder inner voice.

I could write a list of things to help you with self-love. I could tell you to stop comparing yourself to others. Or not to let yourself be defined by what everyone else thinks of you. Logically, we know that this kind of thinking isn't the path to happiness. Unfortunately, knowing something doesn't stop us from suffering the lack of confidence and second-guessing that comes with "ugly days". Often, underlying emotions and past experiences contribute to us living with a lack of self-love on a day-to-day basis.

Over the last three weeks, we've built some new habits into your routine. Big or small, each of these habits will help you rediscover and amplify self-love. Yes, there will still be days when you fall out of love with yourself. Just try and come back to these positive actions as a way of reminding yourself to be kinder and less judgemental.

Ageing and Self-love

Our face is how we're recognized by the outside world and is a huge part of our self-identity. No wonder it freaks us out when we see it ageing before our very eyes! Remember that you are not your face; your face is *part of you*. You are so much more than how you appear to the outside world. Ageing is a gift and is the one sure thing in life that unites us.

Gratitude

I am thankful and appreciate my amazing body.
I am grateful for my health, my family, my work, my passion, my friends.
Something that made me smile this week was …
When I look at my body, I am grateful for …
I am grateful for this new day.

Happiness

Positivity is a choice. I choose to be positive.

Affirmations

I accept and love myself unconditionally.
I am proud of what I have achieved and how far I've come.
When I look at myself in the mirror, I know that I love, and I am loved.
I'm unique. I don't compare myself to others.
I value myself. I value my mind, my emotions, my body and my spirit.
I am mindful of my thoughts because my thoughts shape my reality.
I choose to act in a way that is kind to myself.

Breathwork

This week we're focusing on a more energizing breathwork with a stimulating exercise called Bellows Breath. It's traditionally used in yoga to help boost energy and stimulate circulation, leaving you feeling re-energized and more focused. It's best to practise first thing in the morning or whenever you need a pick-me-up.

1. You might want to blow your nose first! Sit upright in a relaxed position. Start to breathe forcefully, in and out through your nose, with your mouth closed. Try and do one breath per second. Imagine you're pushing the breath out of your nose with as much strength as you can – a bit like a snort.

2. Repeat this for twenty seconds. Make sure you're breathing from your diaphragm and that your belly is softly moving. Once you've finished the twenty-second cycle, rest for up to one minute while breathing normally, then repeat.

3. If you start to feel light-headed, take a moment to rest while breathing naturally, then once you're feeling back to normal, try it again at a slower, less intense pace. As you get more comfortable with this practice, you can start to do it for longer, working up to sixty seconds.

Physical Support

In week 3, we learnt how to use gua sha on your face. This week, we'll take it down onto the body.

We'll be aiming to ease tension in your muscles while stimulating blood flow and lymphatic flow. As you glide, you might find areas of tension.

You can use a gua sha on your body without any lubricant. However, this can drag the skin. I think gua shas work best in tandem with water or oil — I like to use mine in the shower. As a general rule, use the inner or outer curve to make long, upward strokes. The inner curve gives a more generalized glide, whereas the outer curve allows for more depth. I prefer working in the direction of the lymphatic system, but you won't do any harm if you do not.

Repeat each glide three to eight times. If you're short on time, do fewer strokes or focus on one part of your body.

It's common to come up pink where you have glided. If you come up with some love bite-like type stripes, that's not a bad thing! You may just want to go lighter and leave it a few days before repeating the moves in this area.

Arms: move from your wrist to your elbow, elbow to shoulder and up toward your armpit.

Thighs: scrape from your knee to your groin in straight lines up, covering your inner, middle, outer and back of your thigh. Avoid scraping over the knee joint.

Lower leg: glide from ankle to knee, in lines.

Buttocks: I like to use the outer curve to glide up and down in rows from the hip to your sit bones.

Lower back: if you can, take both arms behind you, holding the gua sha in your hands. Using the outer curve, glide down from your scapular to your sacrum, one side of the spine then the other. Avoid the spine itself.

Sacrum: glide over the sacrum area (be careful, as it's bony) making smaller, shorter strokes.

Stomach: using light pressure and the inner curve, glide down in rows from under your ribs to your pelvis. Wait several hours after eating before using your gua sha here.

Shoulders: lift your arm and rest your hand on the opposite shoulder. Using your other hand, glide up and down the sides of the trapezius muscle and backs of the deltoids.

Neck and shoulders: I find that the inner curve glides easily in this area. However, most of us hold a lot of tension in the neck and shoulders. If this is the case, the outer curve can be great for working a little deeper. Glide down and out from the occipital across the top of the trapezius.

Feet: it's also really nice to use the outer curve on the soles of your feet.

Physical Activity

In my late teens and early twenties, I was always the first person on the dancefloor and the last one off. My friends and I would drive miles around the country to go to clubs, raves and events, just to dance for hours on end. I've also danced with my kiddies throughout their lives. When they were babies, we'd do kitchen dancing; as they got to be teenagers, I'd go to gigs with them.

I've never had a professional lesson in anything like salsa, ballet or ballroom. But it's never too late to start – and my mother took up flamenco dancing in her forties! One of the things I love about dancing is that you don't **need** lessons. Just throw on some music and move your limbs – there are no rules. It's also probably the fastest way to boost your mood – and it's free. When I've been sitting at my desk for hours, nothing beats getting up and throwing some moves.

Dancing is used as a therapy, and there are many scientifically proven benefits:

- improves coordination

- improves posture and flexibility

- boosts mood

- increases muscular strength

- boosts blood flow

This week, I want you to choose some of your favourite tunes and dance. Inside, outside, in a field – wherever takes your fancy. Switch it up as you go through the week by dancing at different times of the day to different styles of music – anything from classic to house, rock, jazz and deep moody tunes. Just dance as if no one is watching. If it makes you feel a bit awkward, start by shaking your body, moving from your feet to your legs, then work up your body to your shoulders, arms and head.

Dance for a minimum of three full minutes every day. Journal how it feels, physically and emotionally, and how the different music impacts the experience and how much it makes you smile.

Nutrition

Hormones play a huge role in our overall wellbeing and the appearance of our skin. It's a complex subject, and there are no quick fixes. However, eating in a way that supports hormonal balance can really benefit our skin – especially for anyone suffering from acne and/or going through menopause.

Foods to add in

Cruciferous vegetables

These contain a compound called Indole-3-carbinol, which supports liver function. As the liver helps regulate hormone levels, it's essential that we get a good supply of this phytonutrient from our diet.

Broccoli
Cauliflower
Brussels sprouts

Cabbage
Kale
Bok choy

Good fats

Essential fats are vital for hormone production and reducing inflammation.

Olive oil
Flaxseed oil
Avocado oil

Avocado
Unsalted nuts and nut butter
Salmon

Phytoestrogens

These are plants that create a similar effect within the body as natural oestrogen. They are particularly vital when oestrogen levels start dropping off as we approach menopause.

Soy
Flaxseeds
Sesame seeds
Berries

Peaches
Oats
Barley
Wheat bran

Protein

Provides essential amino acids for repair and helps control the hormones that govern appetite.

Chicken	Chickpeas
Eggs	Lentils
Fish	Quinoa
Tofu	Peas

Wholegrains

These give us much-needed B vitamins, which help support the elimination of spent hormones and reduce PMS.

Buckwheat	Oatmeal
Brown rice	(Pop)corn
Bulgar wheat	

Magnesium

Magnesium helps support healthy thyroid function, reduces adrenalin and cortisol, increases serotonin and balances oestrogen.

Pumpkin seeds	Kale
Almonds	Squash
Tuna fish	Kiwi
Spinach	Papaya
Swiss chard	

Vitamin N: Barefoot Walking and Grounding

When did you last walk barefoot outside? As kids, we did this all the time. These days, most of us are lucky if we do it a couple of times a year on a beach. This week, we're going to make barefoot walking a regular thing. There are many benefits for health – particularly our emotional wellbeing. There's also some scientific research supporting the positive effects of "grounding". You can walk on grass, mud or sand – the most important thing is to allow your skin to touch the ground. Walk around for a few minutes, in the sunshine, rain, wind or snow – no excuses! Notice and enjoy the sensation of the soles of your feet on the ground as you take the time to look around at your surroundings.

The science of grounding

If you haven't heard of grounding (also known as "earthing"), it essentially means walking barefoot on the earth. Our bodies have electrical conductivity, and the earth acts like a large battery that balances and recharges our bodies. And as we walk on the earth in bare feet, our bodies pick up free ions from the earth's surface, which act as antioxidants. Most shoes today have rubber soles. As rubber acts as an insulator, it prevents our body from receiving the free ions, so we're unable to reap the benefits.

One eight-week study found that a daily grounding practice improved sleep quality and reduced stress levels among the participants.[133] Beyond that, it has also been linked to a decrease in inflammation, faster wound healing, reduced anxiety and more energy.

Deep Dive: How are Wrinkles Formed?

Wrinkle formation is more than just skin deep. We have wrinkles that are formed as a result of collagen and elastin degradation. Then we have wrinkles which are created by muscle and tissue contraction. The latter "dynamic wrinkles" appear as lines in the skin overlying contracted muscles (such as on your forehead). These wrinkles are always in the opposite direction (perpendicular) to the muscle fibres. They're also mostly connected to our facial expressions. So, they're *a good* thing – no one wants an expressionless face!

My tips to reduce wrinkles:

- sleep on your back

- wear SPF daily

- use a night-time retinoid

- don't smoke

- cut back on sugar

- massage your face daily

- wear dark glasses when it's sunny to prevent squinting

- focus on relaxation methods – frowning and stress shows in more ways than one

Skincare

Let's revisit the importance of the shoulder stretches and warm-up moves we learnt in weeks 1 and 2, to help release muscle tension. Frown lines or eleven lines are often there due to stress, tension, pain and deep concentration. When we are relaxed emotionally we are less likely to be frowning.

From now on we are going to add in some specific evening frown-line massage moves daily. I would like you to include the forehead moves 4, 5 and 6 as a daily practice, alongside your other core methods.

Face Massage: Forehead and Scalp

When thinking about the forehead, there are two main areas we need to consider: lines going across the forehead and frown lines between the brows (eleven lines). There are also different types of wrinkles caused by different muscles.

Lines going across the forehead horizontally are caused by the action of the frontalis muscle, which contracts to raise our eyebrows. It also works to create a variety of different facial expressions: a single brow raised in surprise or an expression that conveys disgust, for example. These movements can cause more of a square or circular wrinkle formation in the middle of the forehead, rather than single lines.

Eleven lines occur between the eyebrows, largely as a result of frowning, concentrating, squinting or being angry. These appear in the glabellar region (the area between your brows) and look like the number eleven.

All these muscle fibres of the forehead area are running in a similar direction, up and down. The frontalis actually has a slight gap as we get to the upper part of the forehead as it divides into two sections.

I've worked on thousands of faces over the years, so know that some people have more of a genetic predisposition to forehead lines than others. Some of us also just happen to have particularly expressive foreheads! Stress, worry, anger (and poor eyesight) all play their part too.

Frown lines are one of the areas I get asked about most. Facial massage can definitely help. But as I've said before, it's not a magic bullet – and will neither prevent lines from forming nor make any existing ones vanish overnight. Anyone who sells you that dream is lying.

The good news is that massage can go a long way to softening expression lines. By stimulating blood flow and lymphatic drainage, it can help create a wide-eyed appearance, making us look happier and more relaxed. Combine massage techniques with the right active ingredients – and even professional treatments – and you'll begin to see a real difference.

If you've had Botox, you can still perform a forehead massage – just make sure you leave a four-week gap after your last appointment. Botox works by preventing the muscles from contracting. So, using massage to boost blood flow in this area is actually very important.

Note: The following moves can be performed on the eyebrows themselves. However, if you're worried about yours falling out, or have had them tattooed, it's fine to work either side of your brows.

···• Forehead Massage •···

Repeat each movement five to eight times.

Start with no oil

1. Place the pads of your fingers along your hairline and make small, firm circles, moving the skin over the bones. Continue to make this movement, covering the whole forehead to release muscle tension. You can also do this movement on your scalp.

2. With your thumb and forefinger (thumb below your brow, finger above), pinch the inner brow, lift and hold. Fake a frown motion and release. Repeat five times.

3. Move your fingers out to the middle of your brow and repeat.

With a small amount of oil

1. Place all your fingers firmly above your brows and push up from your brow to your hairline. Repeat five times.

2. Zigzag your fingers across the entire brow area, using one or two fingers.

3. Place one finger under one brow. Following the curve of your brow, lift upward. Use your free hand to rub from side to side on the lifted area above the brow. Repeat on the other brow.

4. Place your hands on your forehead, with your fingers pointing down toward your brows. Finger walk over your forehead lines, gently lifting and smoothing as you go. Do the same movement on your eleven lines.

5. Repeat this movement, moving up the middle of the forehead toward your hairline.

6. With your fingers in the same position (pointing downward), place your fingers on your frown lines, lift and hold for a count of five, separating your fingers slightly as you do so. Place your fingers slightly higher and repeat. Do the same thing at your hairline.

WITH OIL

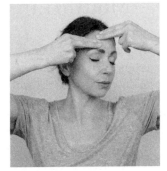

2.

NO OIL

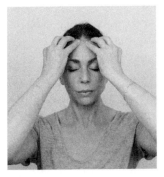

1.

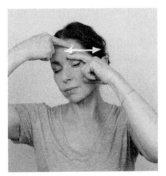

3.

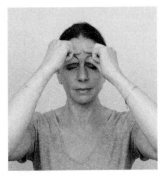

2.

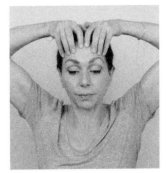

4.

···· This Week's Target Area: ····
Mouth/Lips/Nasolabial Lines

A key point to note here is the direction of your facial muscles. Sometimes we need to work *across* them – rather than in the same direction – in order to get the best results.

1. Pinch lift: place one finger under your eyes either side of your nose, with your thumbs on your jawline either side of your mouth. Glide your thumbs up to your fingers. Hold, lift and snarl.

2. Repeat the last move but make it smaller, working from your nostrils up as you move out across your face.

3. Support the side of your mouth. Make flicking movements with the other hand, moving along the full length of the nasolabial line.

4. Push your tongue into the nasolabial line from the inside of your mouth, and repeat the above move.

5. Extend this movement by using all your fingers to firmly lift the nasolabial line, then hold. Support your lips with your other hand.

6. Finger walk along the nasolabial line.

7. Using two fingers on either side of your mouth, push up from your jaw to your nose using lighter pressure.

8. Place the flat of your finger along the nasolabial fold (both sides at the same time). Flick up and out.

TARGET: MOUTH/LIPS/NASOLABIAL LINES

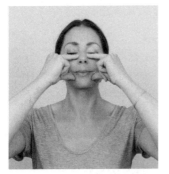

1.

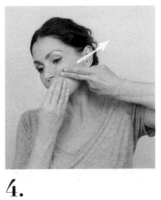

4.

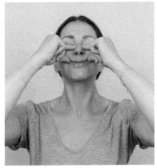

2.

5.

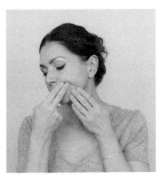

3.

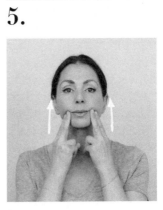

7.

9. Support the side of your nose with the fingers of one hand. Using two fingers from the other hand, pull, flick and glide the skin out and up (working across the muscles).

10. Use your forefingers to work across the muscles of the chin, making small, firm glides in a pulling-apart motion. Cover the whole chin, staying close to the lower lip. Continue this move across your upper lip.

Deep Focus: Buccal Massage

Buccal massage is a method that's been around for decades. Thanks to social media, it has recently become popular again. Buccal involves using your thumb and fingers to massage inside and outside of your mouth and cheeks. It's particularly effective for those wanting to soften facial expression lines on the lower face, re-contour the nasolabial area, ease TMD (temporomandibular disorder) and relieve sinus discomfort.

I first trained in this method over ten years ago. Happily, we can simplify it and build it into our home routine. Just don't be overly aggressive with your movements. As you'll be working on and inside your own face and mouth, you can perform Buccal without surgical gloves. You'll need a simple, non-aromatherapy oil such as rosehip seed, almond, coconut, olive or sea buckthorn. Just the tiniest amount (two to three drops) is enough.

Apply oil to your lower face, mouth, chin and cheeks, and then repeat each of the following movements three times. On exercises that ask you to put your thumb in your mouth, make sure to purse your lips around your thumb in an "O" shape, then soften your mouth and repeat the moves.

As a general rule, the finger that's on the outside of your face will glide toward your lips. You can and will feel lumps and bumps in the tissue. Don't worry – this is totally normal.

TARGET: MOUTH/LIPS/NASOLABIAL LINES

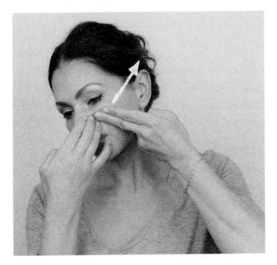

9.

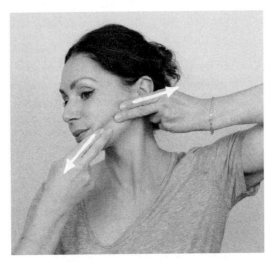

10.

1. Place your thumb inside your mouth. Let your first and second fingers rest on the skin beside your mouth on the outside. Tighten your lips around your thumb and create a gliding "C" shape around one half of your mouth. Push with your thumb and press with your fingers. Glide back and forth, around your orbicularis oris muscle.

2. With your fingers and thumb in the same position, keep your thumb still as you glide your fingers toward your thumb in short strokes. Continue as you work around the side of your mouth. Keep your lips tight around your thumb.

3. The path you should be following is: glide from the side of your nose over the nasolabial area. Then glide from the outer corner of your eye to your mouth. Glide from your ear to your mouth; then your cheek to your mouth; from your jaw to your mouth and from your chin to your lower lip.

4. Place your thumb further inside your mouth and repeat the last move, but now with your thumb and fingers gliding together. Imagine they're stuck together like magnets as they trace along the same path. Keep your lips tight around your thumb in an "O" shape.

5. Use three fingers on the outside of your face to mirror the movement of your thumb inside your mouth as you glide them all from your ear to your mouth.

6. With your thumb still inside your mouth, use your first finger to glide in a curve (imagine you're sucking your thumb and rubbing your skin with your first finger). This movement is more of a rubbing motion.

7. Work around the nasolabial area in this fashion, gliding your bent finger across the skin toward your thumb.

8. Repeat these moves on the other side of your face.

BUCCAL MASSAGE

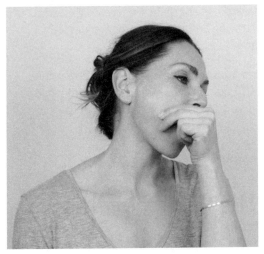

1.

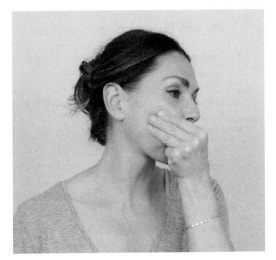

5.

···· Walrus tusks ····

1. Place both thumbs inside your mouth. Glide both of your first fingers in an inward curving glide, like creating a semi-circle on each side, tracing and rubbing over the nasolabial line and upper lip area.

2. Place your first fingers inside your mouth and repeat the move, this time with your thumbs gliding in a semi-circle around the sides of your mouth, from your nose to your chin and back.

⁺⁺ Gadget Highlight: Needling ⁺⁺

I discussed microneedling in more detail on page 199.

My tips for needling:

- Microneedling is best done in the evening on freshly cleansed skin.

- You can exfoliate the skin first with an AHA tonic or wash.

- Used alone, your derma-roller will give your skin a gentle but effective boost. You can also apply a specialized serum before and/or after to amplify results.

- Please avoid using perfumed and creamy serums. Stick to well-formulated cosmeceutical or single-ingredient serums. A hyaluronic acid is a safe and effective choice.

WALRUS TUSKS

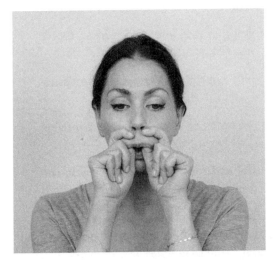

1.

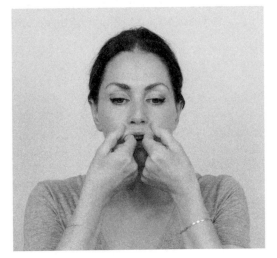

2.

- You can roller with retinoids, but take care. If your skin feels more sensitive than usual, go back to using a hyaluronic acid serum.

- Keep the roller going in one line of direction. Don't turn corners or you risk scratching the skin surface.

- Roll back and forth over the skin without pressing down into it.

- Repeat five to eight times on each area before moving to the next.

- Rolling on the forehead can make you sneeze as the needles work across certain nerve endings!

- Don't massage over freshly needled skin – it will be too stimulating and irritate. Either massage beforehand or massage in the morning. Then needle in the evening.

- Don't overdo it. Start once a week, then gradually increase to a maximum of three times weekly.

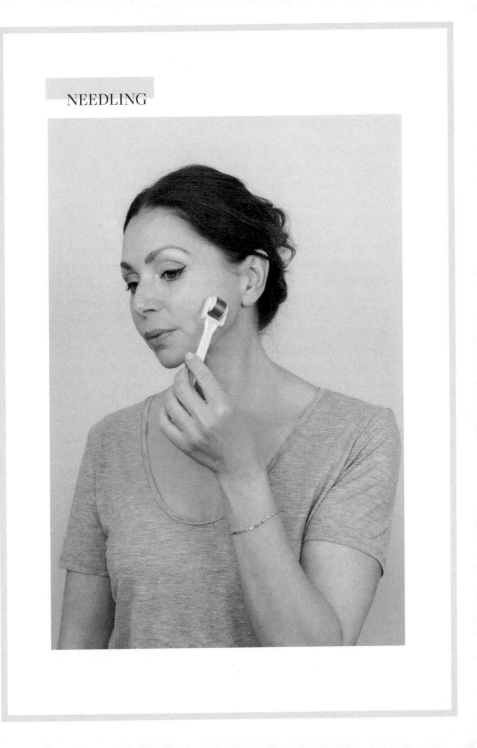

Silver Light Shower Meditation

There are two different methods of using this meditation practice. I like to use each one at different times of the day.

1. Every time you take a shower, imagine there's silver light coming out of the showerhead. Picture it washing over your skin, flowing down your body and rinsing away any negative thoughts, stress, worries, aches and pains. Think of all that negativity washing down the drain.

2. Lie or sit comfortably. Soften your jaw and relax your shoulders. Imagine you're standing underneath a showerhead. Instead of water, a healing silver light is raining down on you. From your head, down to your toes, covering every inch of your skin. Imagine this silver energy running inside your body, through your heart, lungs, stomach, liver, kidneys, bladder and reproductive organs. Picture it purifying, calming, cleansing and healing as the silver light passes through and over your body.

Journalling

1. Three things that I love about myself are …

2. One activity that brings me joy is …

3. I can best nourish and nurture myself when I feel run down by …

4. Three compliments I have received that made me smile are … and this week, I will pay <name> a genuine compliment for …

5. Looking back over the past ten years, I am most proud of …

6. Five years from now, I would like to …

Congratulations – you've completed the plan!

Now's the time to celebrate your achievements, because you've come a long way. Remember that success is not just about an end goal, but about making baby steps every day.

Some space for your thoughts

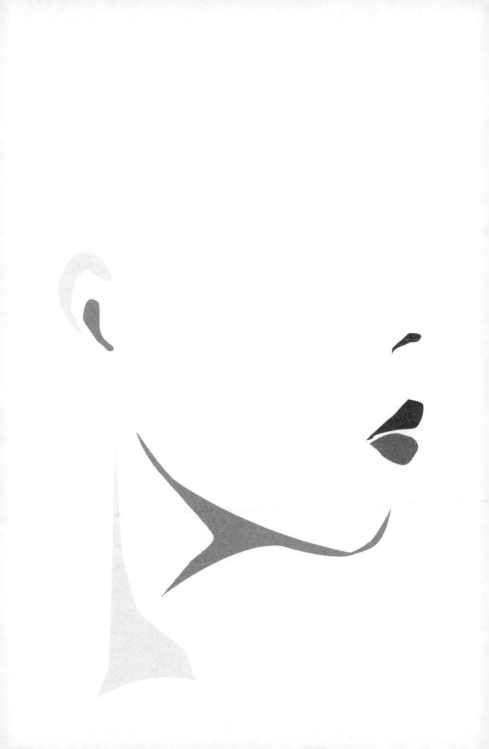

13

After the Plan – What Now?

So, you've completed the four-week plan – congratulations! Now might be a good time to reflect on what you've found most challenging, most easy – and most transformative.

The plan is intended to give you a boost and kick-start some healthy habits. But, what now? The short answer is: rinse and repeat! It might not be possible for you to complete all the actions every single day forever, but now's the time to make a plan going forward, so you stick to the ones you found most valuable. Keep in mind that if you ever feel off-kilter or are going through a particularly tough time, the plan is always here for you to return to when you need to reset and remind yourself that self-care is essential.

Notes

1   www.consumer.healthday.com/encyclopedia/aging-1/age-health-news-7/aging-and-stress-645997.html
2   www.onlinelibrary.wiley.com/doi/abs/10.1111/bjd.17605
3   Hay RJ, Johns NE, Williams HC et al. The global burden of skin disease in 2010: an analysis of the prevalence and impact of skin conditions. J Invest Dermatol 2014; 134:1527–34
4   www.ncbi.nlm.nih.gov/pmc/articles/PMC3798372/
5   www.apa.org/monitor/2015/02/cover-skin
6   www.piedmont.org/living-better/why-routines-are-good-for-your-health
7   www.growthengineering.co.uk/endorphins-help-you-learn-better/
8   www.positivepsychology.com/benefits-of-journalling/
9   www.psychcentral.com/lib/the-health-benefits-of-journalling#1
10 www.health.harvard.edu/healthbeat/giving-thanks-can-make-you-happier
11 www.ft.com/content/0a8d56f8-6111-4829-9730-95ef2ddeff8f
12 https://alertatwork.com/understanding-time-preference-as-a-diversity-issue/
13 www.sleepfoundation.org/physical-health/cancer-and-sleep
14 www.bostonmagazine.com/health/2013/11/18/why-heart-attacks-happen-morning/
15 www.apa.org/news/press/releases/stress/2013/sleep
16 www.apa.org/news/press/releases/stress/2013/sleep
17 www.time4sleep.co.uk/blog/happy-positive-and-motivated-why-good-sleepers-are-content-in-their-careers
18 www.sleepeducation.org/news/2015/07/24/how-sleep-deprivation-ages-you-quicker
19 www.mdedge.com/dermatology/article/233377/aesthetic-dermatology/circadian-rhythms-does-time-day-you-use-skin-care?sso=true
20 www.byrdie.com/beauty-sleep
21 www.medicalnewstoday.com/articles/318996#Activity-of-skin-protecting-enzyme-altered
22 www.pubmed.ncbi.nlm.nih.gov/20678867/
23 www.skinshop.co.uk/skinmagazine/can-lack-of-sleep-trigger-eczema
24 www.medicalnewstoday.com/articles/how-gut-microbes-contribute-to-good-sleep
25 www.ncbi.nlm.nih.gov/pmc/articles/PMC6950569/
26 www.sciencedaily.com/releases/2020/02/200220141731.htm
27 www.sleepfoundation.org/children-and-sleep/how-blue-light-affects-kids-sleep
28 www.nutraingredients-usa.com/Article/2020/10/12/Ashwagandha-s-sleep-benefits-to-extend-to-people-with-insomnia-RCT

29 www.healthline.com/health/gamma-aminobutyric-acid#side-effects
30 www.forbes.com/sites/alicegwalton/2015/02/09/7-ways-meditation-can-actually-change-the-brain/?sh=518ea42f1465
31 www.elitedaily.com/p/why-meditation-makes-you-happy-according-to-science-8333117
32 www.mayoclinic.org/tests-procedures/meditation/in-depth/meditation/art-20045858
33 www.health.harvard.edu/blog/mindfulness-meditation-helps-fight-insomnia-improves-sleep-201502187726
34 https://www.youtube.com/channel/Abigailjames1
35 www.yogauonline.com/yoga-therapy-training/integrative-restoration-yoga-nidra-and-veterans-ptsd
36 www.ncbi.nlm.nih.gov/pmc/articles/PMC6134749/
37 www.webmd.com/sleep-disorders/pink-noise-sleep
38 www.independentliving.co.uk/advice/too-much-sitting-down/
39 www.ncbi.nlm.nih.gov/pmc/articles/PMC4838429/
40 www.health.harvard.edu/staying-healthy/exercising-to-relax
41 www.healthline.com/health/depression/exercise#Exercise-and-brain-chemistry
42 www.pdb101.rcsb.org/motm/162
43 www.everydayhealth.com/skin-beauty/the-scientific-reasons-why-exercise-can-give-you-better-looking-skin/
44 www.ucsf.edu/news/2013/09/108886/lifestyle-changes-may-lengthen-telomeres-measure-cell-aging
45 www.annualreviews.org/doi/abs/10.1146/annurev-physiol-020518-114310
46 www.ncbi.nlm.nih.gov/pmc/articles/PMC4531076
47 www.youthandearth.com/blogs/blog/ampk-longevity-pathway
48 www.lifeextension.com/magazine/2018/ss/turn-on-your-bodys-youth-switch
49 www.ncbi.nlm.nih.gov/pmc/articles/PMC2779044/
50 www.nationaleczema.org/eczema-exercise/
51 www.canr.msu.edu/news/walking_helps_prevent_chronic_disease
52 www.www.heart.org/HEARTORG/HealthyLiving/PhysicalActivity/Walking/Walk-Dont-Run-Your-Way-to-a-Healthy-Heart_UCM_452926_Article.jsp#.WaWZw_nyuHs
53 www.ncbi.nlm.nih.gov/pubmed/27100368
54 www.apa.org/pubs/journals/releases/xlm-a0036577.pdf
55 www.ncbi.nlm.nih.gov/pubmed/27100368
56 www.nature.com/articles/s41430-020-0558-y
57 www.globalwellnesssummit.com/2019-global-wellness-trends/prescribing-nature/
58 www.webmd.com/lung/news/20201231/get-out-nature-is-the-fix-for-covid-19-stress
59 www.ncbi.nlm.nih.gov/pmc/articles/PMC2820143/

60 www.thethirty.whowhatwear.com/yoga-for-glowing-skin/slide4

61 www.embryo.asu.edu/pages/edgar-allen-and-edward-doisys-extraction-estrogen-ovarian-follicles-1923

62 www.ncbi.nlm.nih.gov/pmc/articles/PMC3772914/#:~:text=In%20estrogen%20deficient%20women%20skin,by%202%25%20per%20postmenopausal%20year.&text=Type%20I%20and%20III%20skin,observed%20in%20post%2Dmenopausal%20women

63 www.ncbi.nlm.nih.gov/pmc/articles/PMC3772914/#:~:text=In%20estrogen%20deficient%20women%20skin,by%202%25%20per%20postmenopausal%20year.&text=Type%20I%20and%20III%20skin,observed%20in%20post%2Dmenopausal%20women

64 www.dermatologytimes.com/view/solution-estrogen-deficient-skin

65 www.ncbi.nlm.nih.gov/pmc/articles/PMC2685269/

66 www.tonyrobbins.com/health-vitality/the-power-of-cold-water/

67 www.ncbi.nlm.nih.gov/pmc/articles/PMC3064898/

68 www.researchgate.net/publication/5854059_Adapted_cold_shower_as_a_potential_treatment_for_depression

69 www.ncbi.nlm.nih.gov/pmc/articles/PMC6766865/#jdv15583-bib-0004

70 www.who.int/health-topics/air-pollution#tab=tab_1

71 www.ncbi.nlm.nih.gov/pmc/articles/PMC6766865/#jdv15583-bib-0004

72 www.blf.org.uk/support-for-you/indoor-air-pollution/about-indoor-air-pollution

73 www.ncbi.nlm.nih.gov/pmc/articles/PMC6766865/#jdv15583-bib-0004

74 www.ncbi.nlm.nih.gov/pmc/articles/PMC6766865/#jdv15583-bib-0004

75 www.ncbi.nlm.nih.gov/pmc/articles/PMC6766865/#jdv15583-bib-0004

76 www.ncbi.nlm.nih.gov/pmc/articles/PMC5446966/

77 www.link.springer.com/article/10.1007/s40257-020-00551-x

78 www.ncbi.nlm.nih.gov/pmc/articles/PMC3869874/

79 www.onlinelibrary.wiley.com/doi/abs/10.1111/jdv.13301

80 www.corneotherapy.org/education/courses-for-non-members

81 www.corneotherapy.org/about-corneotherapy/science-of-corneotherapy

82 www.paulaschoice.com/ingredient-dictionary/thickeners%2Femulsifiers/emulsifier.html

83 www.corneotherapy.org/articles/226-emulsifiers-in-skin-care

84 www.paulaschoice.co.uk/alcohol-in-skincare-the-facts

85 www.todayswoundclinic.com/articles/nutritional-factors-wound-healing-older-adult-patient

86 www.paulaschoice.co.uk/amino-acids-hydrate-skin

87 www.lpi.oregonstate.edu/mic/health-disease/skin-health#reference32

88 www.lpi.oregonstate.edu/mic/health-disease/skin-health/vitamin-C

89 www.nuffieldhealth.com/article/how-to-make-your-own-vitamin-d-face-mask

90 www.pubmed.ncbi.nlm.nih.gov/10594744/

91 www.lpi.oregonstate.edu/mic/health-disease/skin-health/vitamin-E

92 www.lpi.oregonstate.edu/mic/health-disease/skin-health/flavonoids

93 www.usgs.gov/special-topic/water-science-school/science/water-you-water-and-human-body?qt-science_center_objects=0#qt-science_center_objects

94 www.sciencedaily.com/releases/2016/11/161117151059.html

95 www.ncbi.nlm.nih.gov/pmc/articles/PMC6985772/

96 www.ncbi.nlm.nih.gov/pmc/articles/PMC6048199/

97 www.aedit.com/aedition/relationship-between-unhealthy-gut-microbiome-skin-conditions

98 https://mplsimc.com/could-your-skin-issues-be-yeast-overgrowth-or-candida/

99 www.self.com/story/what-niacinamide-can-do-for-your-skin

100 www.pubmed.ncbi.nlm.nih.gov/27548886/

101 www.ncbi.nlm.nih.gov/pmc/articles/PMC5522662/

102 www.pubmed.ncbi.nlm.nih.gov/20646083/

103 www.medicalnewstoday.com/articles/fish-oil-for-skin#dry-skin-and-eczema

104 www.renewalliance.com/blogs/i/collagen-supplement-facts-and-myths

105 www.drruscio.com/research-show-marine-collagen/

106 www.elle.com/uk/beauty/skin/a28644116/magnesium-benefits/

107 www.pubmed.ncbi.nlm.nih.gov/32083522/

108 www.hollandandbarrett.com/the-health-hub/vitamins-and-supplements/supplements/what-is-silica/

109 www.byrdie.com/silica-benefits

110 www.womanandhome.com/beauty/beauty-news/average-woman-spends-skincare-321315/

111 www.telegraph.co.uk/beauty/face/87-per-cent-women-confused-skincare-products-ultimate-simple/

112 www.ncbi.nlm.nih.gov/pmc/articles/PMC5796020/

113 www.patient.info/news-and-features/does-spf-moisturiser-give-you-enough-sun-protection

114 www.netdoctor.co.uk/beauty/skincare/a28090/how-skin-affects-confidence/

115 https://ziipbeauty.com/abigail20

116 Watch my preferred microneedling technique here: www.youtube.com/watch?v=EJknmsrgMN8

117 www.nursingtimes.net/clinical-archive/dermatology/skin-1-the-structure-and-functions-of-the-skin-25-11-2019/

118 www.medicalnewstoday.com/articles/262881

119 www.venustreatments.com/en-gl/blog/what-is-elastin-the-beauty-benefits-of-elastic-fibers/

ABOUT THE AUTHOR

120 www.byrdie.com/benefits-of-facial-massage-4690049
121 www.ncbi.nlm.nih.gov/books/NBK519014/
122 www.ncbi.nlm.nih.gov/books/NBK519014/
123 www.healthline.com/health/how-many-times-do-you-blink-a-day
124 www.psychologytoday.com/gb/blog/urban-survival/201505/5-ways-stress-hurts-your-body-and-what-do-about-it
125 www.livescience.com/35332-face-bones-aging-110104.html
126 www.ncbi.nlm.nih.gov/books/NBK551530/
127 www.florida-academy.edu/history-of-massage-therapy/
128 www.amcollege.edu/blog/dutch-origins-of-swedish-massage-amc-miami
129 www.harpercollins.com/blogs/authors/kundan-mehta
130 www.m-t-n.co.uk/kobido-japanese-face-massage/
131 www.shawellnessclinic.com/en/shamagazine/look-younger-with-kobido-facial-massage/
132 www.thelymphoedemacliniclondon.co.uk/pages/manual-lymphatic-drainage.php
133 www.ncbi.nlm.nih.gov/pmc/articles/PMC4378297/

About the Author

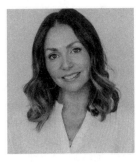

Abigail James is a multi-award winning advanced facialist and wellbeing expert with 20 years of hands-on industry experience and numerous qualifications to her name. She is known worldwide for her extensive knowledge, facial massage and results-driven bespoke treatments.

Referred to in the press as "The Queen of Skin" and "the Priestess of facial massage", Abigail was one of the original trailblazers for a combined approach to skin health, combining beauty, nutrition and mental health with nature, science, technology and hands-on skills. She has worked within the spa and skincare industry, both in her own private London clinics and global locations, private members clubs and retreats. Abigail is a regular industry awards judge and consults to luxury skincare and lifestyle brands. Some of her treatment designs and menus can be found in five-star hotels around the world. She contributes and features extensively in the media and has been spokesperson and in-house advisor to numerous brands. Abigail has a loyal clientele and ever-growing global following on social media.

Youtube: @AbigailJames
Instagram: @Abigailjames
Website: Abigailjames.com
Blog: The Beauty Breakfast Blog

The Glow Plan is Abigail's second book. Her first book, *Love your Skin*, published in 2017.

"Ageing is a gift" - Abigail James

Acknowledgements

Firstly I need to thank my clients and followers; you guys inspire me daily to try to be the best I can be, to continue my learning to be able to better support and share my knowledge and skills physically in treatment and online with you.

Thank you to my kiddies, Georgia, James and Reuben for being my biggest cheerleaders (in a yeah you're just our mum, teenager kinda way). You are my driving force, my team of diamond shaped rocks.

Thank you to Adrian at Kruger Cowne for helping turn my ideas into books. Bella Blissett, for your simply amazing ability to turn my words into something amazing and to the team at Watkins for allowing me the freedom to create this book in the format you see, specifically Fiona Robertson and Anya Hayes.

Thank you to Nichola Moore for your incredible nutritional knowledge and to Sarah Fretwell for your beautiful yogi words and vibes. Dan Roberts, your turn next dude!

I also wanted to say thank you to Charles, for listening to all the crazy ideas and support.

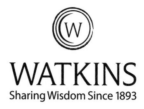

WATKINS

Sharing Wisdom Since 1893

The story of Watkins began in 1893, when scholar of esotericism John Watkins founded our bookshop, inspired by the lament of his friend and teacher Madame Blavatsky that there was nowhere in London to buy books on mysticism, occultism or metaphysics. That moment marked the birth of Watkins, soon to become the publisher of many of the leading lights of spiritual literature, including Carl Jung, Rudolf Steiner, Alice Bailey and Chögyam Trungpa.

Today, the passion at Watkins Publishing for vigorous questioning is still resolute. Our stimulating and groundbreaking list ranges from ancient traditions and complementary medicine to the latest ideas about personal development, holistic wellbeing and consciousness exploration. We remain at the cutting edge, committed to publishing books that change lives.

DISCOVER MORE AT:
www.watkinspublishing.com

Read our blog

Watch and listen to
our authors in action

Sign up to
our mailing list

We celebrate conscious, passionate, wise and happy living.

Be part of that community by visiting

 /watkinspublishing   @watkinswisdom

▶ /watkinsbooks   ⊡ @watkinswisdom